MENOPAUSE
A TIME FOR POSITIVE CHANGE

MENOPAUSE

A TIME FOR POSITIVE CHANGE

Judi Fairlie, Jayne Nelson
and Ruth Popplestone

BLANDFORD PRESS

POOLE · NEW YORK · SYDNEY

First published in the UK 1987 by Blandford Press
Link House, West Street, Poole, Dorset BH15 1LL

Distributed in Australia by
Capricorn Link (Australia) Pty Ltd
PO Box 665, Lane Cove, NSW 2066

British Library Cataloguing in Publication Data

Fairlie, Judi
   Menopause: a time for positive change.
   1. Menopause
   I. Title II. Nelson, Jayne
   III. Popplestone, Ruth
   612'.655   RG186
       ISBN 0 7137 1721 1

Printed and bound in Great Britain by
Biddles Ltd, Guildford.

CONTENTS

INTRODUCTION

We are three women: one of 49 who is approaching the menopause; one of 48 who has had her menopause; and one of 47 who hasn't yet started her menopause. When we began trying to learn about the menopause, we all discovered how little is really known about it, and how few good books or pamphlets there are around for women like ourselves who are interested and want to know more. Very few writers encouraged women to help themselves and take responsibility for their own health care as far as possible.

Some of the information we found contained misleading statements, negative attitudes towards women and the menopause, and did not seem to be about real women.

The few books and pamphlets that were available were mostly written from a man's point of view about women's bodies, even some of those written by women. They were often medical or scientific in tone and talked about the menopause as if it were a deficiency disease or illness, rather than a natural event. They promoted the idea that women need drugs and medical assistance, rather than enlightened self-help. Some writers made quite frightening statements, which have never really been satisfactorily proved or challenged, about the occurrence or severity of symptoms which they claim are caused by the menopause.

Much of the information we found had cold, clinical statistics and complicated diagrams which only looked at the gynaecological 'bits' of women so that it was often hard to know where in the body they actually belonged. These strange fragments of bodies seemed to have nothing to do with us as whole, warm, living, individual women.

In Britain, there is a stigma attached to the menopause, and this is nourished and kept alive by the many myths and jokes about the menopause, and menopausal women. We found that many of the books or pamphlets used stereotypes to illustrate their points; for example, there was the idea of *all* women being 'housewives' with children and a businessman husband who is the breadwinner.

These categorised views tell us nothing about real women; but they do tell us a lot about the massive ignorance amongst many doctors and specialists about the changing realities of women's lives. They also show extreme insensitivity to many of the women who are their patients or who might read their information.

For all these reasons, we wanted to write this book to share with other women what we have found out about the menopause; to share ideas on what we can do to try to be responsible for our own health in our middle or older years; to see how we can challenge the negative attitudes, myths and stereotypes attached to the menopause and older women so that they don't damage or interfere with our *own* experiences of menopause or middle age; and to suggest ideas as to how we can make the menopause a positive time of life for ourselves.

We have tried to make this book useful to *all* women regardless of race, class and sexuality, and to be aware of attitudes we have expressed which might be offensive to other women. However, there are gaps in the knowledge available: for instance little has been collected and shared about the experience of menopause from lesbian women, and women from ethnic minority groups who live in Britain. We would therefore welcome any comments which would make future editions of this book more relevant.

ABOUT THE AUTHORS

JUDI FAIRLIE

I am a full-time lecturer in a Further Education College, running an Access Course for mature students, and teaching biology. I married for a second time three years ago. Two of my sons are still living at home, two other sons and a daughter have moved away to work. I was a single parent for ten years, but was fortunate that I was able to share the care of the children with their father. In 1972–77 I lived in the East End of London in the first GLC tenants cooperative.

My interest in the menopause was triggered off when I missed a period three years ago. As I was in my forties I wondered if I had started my menopause. In fact at the time I was moving house and job and getting married again – later when things settled down my periods returned. I decided to follow up my interest in the menopause when I took an MSc in Health Education. I was 45 when I was accepted as a mature student to do the MSc course. For my dissertation I talked to many women about the menopause and was left in the end with a strong feeling that it was aspects of the lives of women in middle age and other people's attitudes which affected them most and not the menopause itself. Near the end of my dissertation I met Jayne and was excited to meet someone else whom I could talk to about the menopause. We exchanged views and ideas. It might have rested there but Jayne was already in contact with Ruth, with the idea of working together on the menopause.

JAYNE NELSON

I am from a farming family (both parents and both sets of grandparents) in the Midlands.

For the last 20 years I have been a single mother, living in London with my three daughters, now all adult and left home. For the last 18 years I have worked as a secretary to support them, and, during that time, have also been active in NALGO, working on women's issues.

I started my menopause when I was 37 following sterilisation after coming off the pill after 13 years. My last period was in 1980 when I was 40.

In 1981, I was accepted as a mature student on an MA in Women's Studies course at Kent University although I had no 'A' levels or first degree. The union (NALGO) supported me and negotiated financial support from my employers, who also agreed to keep my job open for me. Whilst doing the course, I decided to work on menopause and ageing for my dissertation, in order to understand better what was happening to my own body. After completing my MA, I returned to my job as a secretary, but developed and ran courses in the evenings on menopause and ageing, to share with other women the information I had gathered for my dissertation.

I met Ruth when I went to one of her menopause workshops, and Judi when she contacted me to discuss my research and courses. The three of us worked on a Menopause Broadsheet for WHIC, and wrote articles for the GLC Women's Committee Bulletin before writing this book together.

In 1981, I moved house, and now live with other women in North London. I have been celibate for a number of years whilst considering my sexuality. I have recently changed jobs from being a secretary to part-time tutor in Adult Education. My mid-life changes have been, and are, sometimes scary, but liberating and exciting. I still continue to have sweats and flushes. I look forward to being in my fifties with great anticipation.

RUTH POPPLESTONE
I was brought up in Kent, studied at Manchester University and then trained to be a social worker. I worked in the Midlands, the North of England and Scotland before returning to the South.

I am divorced and now live with a friend in London.

I job-share a Training Officer post with another woman in an inner London borough. I also work freelance, mainly running training courses and workshops for women.

I met Jayne when she came on one of my menopause workshops.

I enjoy working in groups and I am grateful to Judi and Jayne for everything I have learned through the experience of writing this book together.

1 · WHAT IS THE MENOPAUSE?

Menopause is a word which means different things to different people. Some think of the menopause as the beginning of ageing, or as a medical condition which needs treatment. Others associate it with a life crisis: either as a joke, or to describe emotions that women and men sometimes experience as they enter their middle years. Perhaps they feel they are saying goodbye to their youth, or dread the idea of ageing, or are experiencing changes in themselves which they find confusing or worrying.

The Latin words which make up the word 'menopause' mean the ending of menstruation. Strictly speaking, menopause means our very last period, but popularly, the word has also come to mean the time leading up to the last period and after it. Sometimes the phrase 'the change of life' is used, and some doctors use the term 'the climacteric'.

For each of us, the menopause is a unique and personal experience which depends a lot on our particular life's circumstances: how we feel about the idea of the menopause and how prepared we are for it. We shall be looking at these ideas later in this book.

THE END OF THE MENSTRUAL CYCLE

Monthly periods usually start in adolescence. The menstrual cycle of hormonal chain reactions of egg production (ovulation) followed by the flow of menstrual blood continues every month, unless interrupted, until menopause approaches. Menopause is part of the menstrual cycle, the final part. The menstrual cycle and menopause are controlled by the hormone (endocrine) system. As we approach the menopause, the levels of hormones connected with the menstrual cycle begin to alter, and we begin to produce less of some and more of others. As a result of these changing quantities of hormones in our bloodstream, we may begin to experience certain reactions, which are known as signs or symptoms of menopause. If you want to know in more detail what happens during menstruation, a good book to read is *Our Bodies Ourselves* (see p.102 for details).

SIGNS OF THE MENOPAUSE

Because we consider the menopause to be a natural event and not a disease or illness, we use the word 'signs' of the menopause instead of 'symptoms'.

There are two groups of signs which most people agree are due to the menopause. The first arises from the effects of changing hormone levels on the heart and blood vessels, e.g. hot flushes, hot or cold sweats, palpitations, and cramps. The second group affects the secretions of the vagina, and the linings of the vagina, bladder and urethra (the tube we pass urine through), and sometimes the nasal passages. This can lead to dry nose, dry or sore vagina, and possible increased risk of genital infections. There are of course other reasons for vaginal dryness, which we will refer to later.

There is a variety of conditions which may or may not be directly related to the menopause but which women may experience in their middle years, before or after their menopause. The first group of these includes mood changes, tiredness, listlessness and depression, and may be due to changing hormone levels, but is more likely to be due to other changes taking place in our lives around the time of the menopause. The second group is fluid retention, bloatedness, and other signs of pre-menstrual tension (PMT) which can continue to occur even after we stop menstruating, usually around the time the period would have occurred. The third group, bone and joint aches and pains, is equally likely to affect men, and is due to the natural ageing process, or wear and tear, or possibly the onset of osteoarthritis which is quite common in both sexes from the late 30s onwards.

In Chapter 9 we offer some self-help and other ideas for dealing with these and other conditions if they occur.

THE ENDOCRINE SYSTEM

The endocrine system is made up of a special part of the brain, called the hypothalamus, and the various hormone-producing glands: the pituitary, the parathyroids, the thyroid, the pancreas, the adrenals, and the ovaries. A variety of hormones is produced by the endocrine glands as well as the sex hormones involved in menstruation and menopause. These hormones enter into many body functions, such as: temperature regulation; the circulatory and digestive systems; growth and development of bone; and our emotions and mood changes.

The pituitary gland governs the adrenal glands which are located above the two kidneys in the back of the abdomen. They produce adrenalin in response to shock or stress situations, enabling us to react very quickly in an emergency. Adrenalin makes the heart beat rapidly. If there is a 'hiccup' in the endocrine system, or if we are under a certain amount of stress, a flood of adrenalin may rush through the body *even* when there has been no obvious external 'shock' or emergency to cause it. The rush of adrenalin itself can bring about panicky feelings, anxiety, breathlessness, make the heart beat very quickly (palpitations), and can bring on a hot flush, or sweating. It is easy to confuse these reactions with menopausal signs.

AGE RANGE WHEN MENOPAUSE CAN OCCUR

The menstrual cycle reaches its peak as far as ovulation (or egg production) is concerned in our late 20s to early 30s. Although we usually continue to menstruate regularly for many more years, we may not necessarily produce an egg each month. Any time from our mid-30s onwards, we may begin to have irregular periods as our hormone levels begin to alter gradually. Menopause, or our last period, can occur anytime from our late 30s to our early 60s. Nearly 25 per cent of women have reached menopause by the time they are 45 years of age; about 40 per cent between the ages of 45 and 49 years, and just over 20 per cent between 50 and 54 years.

The wide variation of the *normal* age range for the menopause to occur is often misrepresented in medical books on the subject. This is because medical science deals in statistics rather than real women, so they usually say things like 'the average age of menopause is 49–50 years'. Because of this rather fixed idea of the age of menopause, many women who experience their menopause earlier or later feel, or are told, that they are abnormal, or 'unusual'. A common experience among women having or starting their menopause before they are 43 years old is to find that it is referred to as a premature menopause. Some women might even find that they are not believed, or are patted on the hand and told 'it can't be the menopause, you are far too young'!

HOW LONG WILL THE MENOPAUSE LAST?

For some women periods end abruptly; others go through a stage of irregular periods when the amount of bleeding is changeable. This can last anywhere from a few months to a few years, and can be a frustrating experience, especially if the possibility of pregnancy adds to the uncertainty. Still other women have a gradual change as periods become lighter and shorter within the usual cycle: some periods may be missed, but if they return the timing will be more or less as they would have been if the periods were occurring regularly.

It helps to keep a track of any changing patterns. It is useful to keep a menstrual calendar (see Appendix 2) or diary to show up any differences in the timing and length of the cycle from month to month. Until you know for sure that your periods have finally stopped you should take contraceptive measures for at least 18 months after your last period, if you are in a situation where you might get pregnant. If you experience pre-menstrual tension (PMT), keeping a menstrual calendar will enable you to know when to expect PMT and to take some action to reduce it. You may still have PMT when your period has been missed, without the usual feeling of relief when the bleeding starts.

For many women the two years or so before periods stop are the most difficult emotionally when the hormone levels are beginning to show more pronounced ups and downs. We may not realise at the time, because we can only look back once the menopause has happened and our periods have finally stopped, and see that we *were* approaching the menopause! This kind of depression or mood change almost always goes when our periods finally stop for good.

After periods have stopped, hot flushes or sweats or both may start, or continue for a time. Hot flushes are not unlike the blushes that are so common in adolescence, and the frequency and pattern vary. Some women in their 60s and 70s still have hot flushes, but they usually continue for about 2–5 years after the periods have stopped.

SURGICAL MENOPAUSE

The removal of both (or occasionally part) of the ovaries from women who have not reached the menopause can bring on a sudden and perhaps early menopause – this is referred to sometimes as a surgical menopause. A hysterectomy, when the operation involves removal of part or all of the uterus, but not the ovaries, may also bring on the menopause or cause menopausal signs like hot flushes and sweats until the blood supply and the tissues around the ovaries recover. Women who have had their ovaries removed before the age of 45 are said to be especially at risk from increased bone loss and are usually offered hormone replacement therapy. In any case good diet, exercise and sunlight are important for bone health.

2 · WHAT THE MENOPAUSE IS NOT!

One of the first myths to dispel is that the menopause is an illness or disease. It is neither of these things, but is a natural event: the final part of the menstrual phase of women's lives. Most women's monthly periods come and go throughout the years with very little trouble or bother. The fact that some women have more troublesome periods does not mean that menstruation *itself* is seen as a disease or illness that *all* women must go through every month: PMT is not called a 'symptom of menstruation'. And so it *should* be with the menopause. Most (but not all) women will experience some signs such as sweats or flushes before or after the menopause (which is their very last period). But these signs of the menopause are usually referred to by doctors and specialists as 'symptoms' of the menopause – as though it were an illness or disease! Perhaps this is because it is assumed that anyone who goes to a doctor or specialist is a 'patient' who is 'ill' with something that is producing 'symptoms'.

There are various other myths and jokes about the menopause and middle-aged women. We hear that it makes us become rampant sex-starved nymphomaniacs; that it turns us off sex completely; that it causes us to shoplift; that it makes us go mad; that it turns us into alcoholics; that it makes us absent-minded; that it makes us grow beards; that it makes us go bald; that it makes us old and wrinkled, etc, etc. You can probably add many more to this list yourself!

The problem with these myths and so-called jokes is that we ourselves can sometimes start believing them without being really aware of it. This can make us dread the menopause. Jokes and stories of this kind make the menopause, and middle-aged women, seem ridiculous or freaky. We may feel almost ashamed if we start having sweats or flushes or other signs that could be part of our menopause, and may try to hide the fact from everyone. We don't want anyone to know we are menopausal because of what people might think about us. Indeed, some women do have difficulty at work with bosses' or colleagues' attitudes if it is known that they are menopausal. This shows that other people believe the myths as well.

Such myths can be very damaging to women: economically if our jobs are threatened, and psychologically as well. The following story shows how a woman was affected when she believed one of these myths.

A woman recently rang us up for advice. She was having irregular periods and felt that she might be starting her menopause, and she wanted to know what the signs were. She was most anxious about the fact that her hair was falling out. She said 'I know this is one of the things that happens to women in their menopause – is there anything I can do to stop it?' After reassuring her that hair falling out was nothing to do with the menopause, further conversation revealed that several members of her family also suffered from the same problem. They had been told they were suffering from a nervous complaint called alopecia which causes hair loss, and that this might be something which runs in their family. In spite of this knowledge, she had felt convinced that *her* hair loss was due to the menopause, because she had always understood that the menopause could make women go bald. She was surprised and relieved to know that this was a myth. Even though she was still left with her hair loss problem, she felt it was less disturbing or embarrassing to suffer from it if it had nothing to do with the menopause!

Another major difficulty with the myths and tales, if we believe them, is that the stress and anxiety we may feel about the menopause may actually make things worse. Trying to hide sweats and flushes may make them happen more often, or more strongly.

We need to have a lot of confidence and feel very good about ourselves to dismiss all the negative ideas and attitudes, and not let them affect us. A step towards helping us to do this is to be able to debunk and see through the myths. For example, contrary to newspaper reports, shoplifting is more often carried out by adolescent boys and men than anyone else, according to crime research figures. Many of the myths aren't really about the menopause at all, but are to do with fear of ageing, or stressful circumstances. These factors can affect men as well as women.

We will now look at the myths concerning sex, ageing and mental illness more closely to show them for the nonsense they really are.

SEX

The myths about women, sex and the menopause are either that we want too much or too little! We know that oestrogen levels in the body are much lower after the menopause but we don't depend on oestrogen for an interest in and an ability to enjoy sex. The menopause should not cause our sexual activity to change dramatically one way or the other. So where does the idea come from that at the menopause women may become 'oversexed' or uninterested?

There are many reasons why a woman may become more, or less, interested in sex. Some women feel a great sense of relief that they no longer have to worry about contraception, and as a result they feel more relaxed about sex. However, in any long-standing relationship, sex may have an all-too-familiar and unsatisfying pattern and the menopause may provide an opportunity to withdraw from it. Sometimes the problem is 'in our own heads' – if we believe the myth that the menopause somehow makes us less attractive. Any middle-aged person may become worried about their sexual attractiveness: it is often the reason for a man seeking a sexual relationship with a much younger woman.

Some middle-aged men become anxious about what they see as their failing sexual prowess (and women can be affected by male partners' anxieties). Myths about menopausal women becoming sexually 'rampant' are more likely to reflect men's fears of middle-aged women's sexual capacities if their own sexual needs are declining. It is ironical that by middle age men often have less interest in sex than when they were younger, while middle-aged women may find their sexual interest and capacities increase, possibly because of a more sensitive genital area, or perhaps freedom from worries about conception.

Communicating to our partner what we enjoy about sex may be difficult. First of all we have to be able to identify the things we find stimulating and sensual and then we have to be able to tell our partners what it is we enjoy. We may never have been used to doing this. Unfortunately, our upbringing often makes us feel guilty or inhibited about touching ourselves and others and developing our sensuality. As girls we were unlikely to have been able to masturbate without feeling a sense of doing something forbidden, and this guilt may still be with us as adult women. Masturbation can be healthy for a whole number of reasons – including the production of natural secretions to moisten the vagina. Sometimes the reduction in vaginal secretions which may follow the menopause can make sex an uncomfortable and even painful experience if we have an insensitive partner, or can't talk about it to them.

A couple who have a good relationship will not find this too much of a problem, because they will be able to adapt their lovemaking to find ways of achieving sexual satisfaction. The most important thing to understand about sex at any age is that everyone's experience is individual and personal.

MENTAL ILLNESS

It is not unusual for people to associate the menopause with madness or mental illness.

In the last century, people who were considered to be mad were either sent away and locked up in an asylum, or kept, sometimes tied up, in a dark corner of the house. It is not surprising that madness was very much feared. Although what we now call 'mental illness' is better understood and more treatable, the fears of becoming mad or mentally ill remain, especially at times when we may feel that we are in danger of breaking down, 'losing our grip' or losing control.

There are a number of different kinds of mental illness. The one which women (unlike men) most often suffer from is depression. Recent studies show that certain events in women's day-to-day lives tend to lead to depression. This is something which many women have been aware of for a long time: there are many aspects of our lives which make us feel depressed.

Contrary to some people's beliefs, menopause does *not* cause us to become mentally unstable. Hormonal changes may cause mood swings, particularly during the lead up to the menopause, and some of the domestic and personal changes which take place in mid-life may make some women depressed. The way women are regarded in this society when they are menopausal makes it surprising that more women do not become depressed at this time of life.

AGEING

To help us debunk the myth that the menopause makes women age, we will briefly describe the human ageing process. Ageing starts in both sexes from infancy! The lens of the eye becomes less elastic from early childhood onwards. By adolescence, eyesight and various other body functions may already have passed their peak and be gradually declining. An important body tissue called collagen which is found in bone and cartilage and which makes up a third of our total body protein becomes increasingly tough and less flexible with age. It changes most rapidly in women and men between the ages of 30 and 50.

From our 30s onwards nerve-muscle co-ordination becomes slower in both sexes, movements are less precise and become more difficult; there is a loss of muscular elasticity (which is why sportspeople usually retire young while they are still at their peak). Muscle shrinkage occurs – especially in under-used or unexercised muscles. As muscle bulk shrinks, the skin above may become slacker and wrinkle in men and women. Skin wrinkling can occur in men and women from 30 onwards. So can hair greying, although this can often be an hereditary 'family' matter.

Hair thinning can also occur in both sexes – but baldness is much more common in men than women. From about 40 to 45 onwards, both sexes can become long-sighted, and suffer from high-tone hearing loss. Short-term memory in both sexes becomes less efficient depending on use, and this can affect the ability to recall things from the long-term memory. Middle-age spread or 'flab' can occur in both men and women from the late 30s onwards depending on diet, life-style and body metabolism. In both sexes there is a gradual decline in the functioning of the organs, and a slowing-down of metabolism. Both sexes suffer to a greater or lesser degree from heart disease, arterial disease, hypertension, arthritis, rheumatism and so forth.

In other words, both sexes age at roughly the same speed and in similar ways. The menopause is an event that occurs at some time during a woman's middle years anywhere from her late 30s to early 60s. It does not cause ageing, nor is it 'the' ageing process. It is a *part* of the whole ageing process that began the day we were born.

It is not just the natural effects of increasing years which affect ageing, but differences in health and life-style resulting from social inequalities – such as differences in income, education, and housing. If we are taught, and can afford to exercise and nourish our bodies properly and regularly, we will maintain them in better shape for a longer period of time. For example, incontinence, which can occur in both sexes at any age if muscle tone is very poor, is known to respond well even in very elderly people to a regime of special exercises and correct diet. It could be prevented from occurring in the first place if we knew how to look after ourselves earlier in life. Inequalities in income, education and housing which may lead to premature or exaggerated ageing have nothing to do with the menopause, but are to do with the culture and politics of our society.

THE MALE MENOPAUSE

IS IT REALLY THE MENOPAUSE?

Men obviously cannot have the menopause in the same way as women because they do not have periods! Hormone changes do take place in men as they age. From adolescence onwards the amount of androgens (male sex hormones) produced by the body begins to drop gradually over a long period of time. As men get older their sperm count begins to drop, although most men retain fertility into old age. In the strict biological sense therefore the male menopause is a myth.

In Chapter 4 we will explore the various mid-life changes which might be taking place around the time of the menopause in women to do with ageing, family situations and perhaps at work. The difficulties men experience in adapting to the same kinds of changes in their lives seems to have given rise to the idea of a male menopause.

Some men experience physical and emotional upsets in mid-life which are severe enough to create depression, impotence and loss of interest in sex, and marked changes in behaviour. The 'menopausal male' may start behaving in what people close to him see as an uncharacteristic fashion. The following quotation highlights negative attitudes towards middle age and the menopause:

... But if you're forty-some, combing hair carefully over the bald spot, getting a bit trendy on ties and shirts, depressed sometimes when sober and pushy with the girls on two or three pints ... then you too, sir, may be showing menopausal symptoms .*

As with the menopause in women the idea of the male menopause is associated with stereotypes and the person who is 'menopausal' is put down, often with jibes and jokes similar to those about the 'mother-in-law'.

HOW MEN DEAL WITH MIDDLE AGE

The majority of men in their 40s and 50s who may be going through changes in their personal lives are subject to the same kinds of anxieties and concerns as women of the same age group. The effect of these changes in middle age sometimes gives rise to a loss of confidence which has been called the 'mid-life crisis'. How men deal with their changing circumstances is an individual matter. Some men respond to their desire to keep looking young by pursuing sexual relationships with women a lot younger than themselves – this may actually accentuate their lowered self-confidence. Other men may become anxious or depressed. Either way it puts a great deal of strain on an established relationship – especially if the two people involved can't talk freely about their worries to each other. A long-standing partnership which has grown stale may be blamed, or both partners may blame *her* menopause for his lack of sexual interest or womanising. This is very stressful indeed for the woman and does nothing to help the man deal with his problem.

The fact that articles and books discuss the male menopause seems to indicate that men are expressing their mid-life anxieties and feelings about themselves more than perhaps they used to. The recognition of a 'mid-life crisis' in men shows us that a woman's biological menopause itself is *not* the cause of emotional difficulties in women either, at this time of life. It is the social, family and financial problems which can affect men *and* women which have to be faced up to. These are not matters which can be solved by prescriptions of hormones or tranquillisers, or by starting a new relationship.

* From *The Male Menopause* by Bowskill and Linacre, Pan 1978.

3 · THE SOCIAL AND CULTURAL BACKGROUND TO MENOPAUSE

As we saw in the previous chapter, there are many false ideas around about the menopause and ageing. If we are to understand our own menopause more clearly, we have to be able to reject these false ideas and replace them with more accurate knowledge about ourselves as women, and the society we live in.

We can start by looking at attitudes towards ageing and older women in our society, to see why many women dread getting older. Some women are really depressed about their 40th birthday, for example, feeling that youth and everything good is behind them and that the future holds very little of interest or value for them – it's 'downhill all the way' from then on.

AGEISM

The word 'ageism' describes discrimination against anyone on grounds of age. It usually affects women more than men. Ageism can start quite early in life for some women: a 10 or 12 year old girl being told she is 'too old' to be a tomboy any more, for example. This sort of attitude is often the reason for girls giving up physical activities and hobbies which would stand them in good stead later in life. More obviously, we see examples of ageism in all those advertisements for secretaries, typists, receptionists or waitresses which say 'must be between 16 and 25'. Such advertisers either want a cheap workforce, or young and, by implication, sexy women around the place.

Another widespread discrimination against women associated with age is the way society treats older women by becoming less interested in them and expecting them to fade away quietly from public view any time after they are 40. This 'disappearance' of older women is very obvious in the media where positive images of vigorous and active older and elderly *men* appear everywhere, often in 'important' and powerful contexts. Grey-haired, or bald, bespectacled, wrinkled, or baggy-eyed, often described or thought of as 'distinguished' or eminent men, they appear daily, in the papers and on television. Frequently, they are shown together with much younger, very glamorous women, for example, presenting the news or in a romantic context.

Rarely do women *of the same age* as these men appear *alongside* them – let alone in a sexual or romantic context with younger men. They are invisible. Unless of course they still look as though they are 25 or 30. It is very unusual to see positive images of older women, to reassure younger and middle-aged women that we will also be valued for ourselves – and not our bodies – as we get older.

In some societies and cultures, older and elderly women are revered or looked up to as people of wisdom: 'elders' who have seen and learned much about life, and are a source of knowledge and wisdom for the younger and middle generations. Unfortunately, this is far from the case in British society, even though after the age of 60–65 there are nearly three times as many women around as men, because women live longer.

The few images of older women that do appear in the media are usually the deliberately sensationalised reports of very elderly women being mugged or raped, or the occasional negative pictures of a group of elderly women sitting passively, watching television or being given tea in a home or day-care centre. Or they are the ridiculed figures of fun as played by the popular television comedians of the day. These are hardly the sort of images of older womanhood to make us feel good about getting older ourselves!

Scenes of groups of older and elderly men out in public places enjoying themselves are such an accepted, and acceptable, normal state of affairs in British society that it doesn't get remarked upon. We see them in the pub, the club or the Working Men's Club, playing/watching darts or snooker, walking the dog, working in the garden or allotment, going to football matches, sitting inside or outside cafés, smoking and chatting etc. By contrast, bingo clubs or Women's Institute branches provoke comment as 'the girls' night out' or the 'old biddies gossipping' over cups of tea, jam-making, or their knitting. Such attitudes are cruel to the women who enjoy bingo, or the WI, and do nothing to encourage those who might be lonely and would benefit from meeting up with other women. Negative attitudes keep women in their homes and off the streets, increasing their invisibility. Newspaper headlines about violent acts against elderly women frighten other older women who do not dare to venture out, particularly after dark. Of course violence against women *is* horrible, particularly so against elderly women. But official figures show that women over 60 are the group least likely to be the victims of violence.

All these attitudes are ageist: discrimination against women on account of age. Some people think that women get a better deal because they retire five years earlier than men. But some employers use this as an excuse for getting rid of women who would still like to work for another five years or so to improve their pension position. And do women ever really retire? Most women carry on cooking, cleaning, shopping and washing as they always have done, until they die or can't do it any longer.

All in all, older women 'don't matter', they are not valued or esteemed in our society (although some older women are of course valued as individuals within the family). This is the kind of future that younger and middle-aged women have to look forward to. It is the effect of ageism, and is the background to the menopause. It is hardly surprising that so many women fear or dread getting older, and see the menopause as the sign that they have begun to do so.

As individuals we women have enormous strength and courage. In spite of what society says, or expects of us, we make our own way through life, on our own terms as far as possible, often by challenging or contradicting the stereotyped ideas of what we *should* be like, or *ought* to be doing.

Many women say that after the age of 40 or so they suddenly feel as though they 'dare' to do or say much more than before: they don't care so much what other people might think, and find that maturity brings them a confidence they never used to have as younger women. Other women are even more positive: they say they feel great about being 40, and are more optimistic about themselves and their lives than ever before.

THE POSITION OF WOMEN IN OUR SOCIETY

The ageism which affects women arises from our position in society compared with men. Most of us have become more aware nowadays of the ways we are less well off, or less well protected than men.

Economically, for example, tax laws assume that all women are looked after by a male breadwinner. Women are less well off with regard to social security, tax, mortgages, pensions and other benefits. Women are paid, on average, only three-quarters of a man's wage for doing the same job, have fewer job possibilities and opportunities, and have to fit their job around their domestic or caring responsibilities. It is assumed that these are their real jobs and that they don't need or want careers or satisfying jobs. This is reflected in the *educational system*, where girls are not encouraged or given the same opportunities as boys. *Culturally* and *socially*, women are still expected to get married and spend most of their time child-raising and child-caring. Those women who don't want to conform to this role find it hard to make their way through life. For those who do conform but also choose to work there are very few work-place nurseries, and maternity leave is inadequate, if it exists at all. *Politics* also reflect women's inferior position in society. Very few women can actually get into politics to have a say on behalf of women, and so male-dominated politics decide on cuts in public spending which affect women particularly. For example, successive governments have refused to spend an adequate amount on cervical smears and breast scans even though cancer of the cervix and breast are major killers of women. But large amounts of money are poured into heart transplant operations.

During the last 10–15 years things have begun to change slowly for the better for women, but the sort of changes in society which will value women more equally with men are very slow. For the majority of us there are still far too many social and cultural attitudes which see us as inferior to men. For example, we must look a certain 'feminine' way if we expect to be treated as 'real' women; we must behave in a certain 'ladylike' way if we want to have the approval of society and the men in our lives – whether male relatives, friends, colleagues or bosses. We can all too often find ourselves responding to what is expected of us. We worry about our figures, or our hair, or our looks, or our clothes, instead of thinking about what *we* really want for ourselves, and want to do with our *own* lives. We find it easier just to get on and do all the chores (often before going out to work, and again when we get back) rather than trying to get others in the family or home to do their share. Or we feel that we mustn't make a fuss or argue but must be pleasant when men behave badly or insultingly to us in the home, in the street, or at work. We often find it really difficult to know what we *do* want for ourselves, and even more difficult to ask for it or insist on it if we are refused. Some women say they find it difficult to get out to a daytime or evening class that they enjoy, for instance, because their husbands or partners disapprove, or won't let them, or because they expect their meals to be ready. Even when other members of the family *do* help out, that's exactly what they see themselves as doing – *helping* the woman with *her* jobs around the house. They don't see it as something they should be doing in any case, especially when the woman is working outside the home to earn or contribute to the family income. Many men expect their women to work *and* keep the house looking as if they were at home cleaning it all day!

LANGUAGE: THE WORDS WE USE

Language is the main way we can converse or communicate with each other and get our ideas, thoughts or messages across. And the more clearly and accurately we use language and words in conversation or writing, the more clearly we will be understood.

Much of everyday language reflects the different attitudes towards grown women compared with grown men: the use of Mr for example for any man regardless of his married or single status, but the use of Miss and Mrs, which insists that women identify themselves as belonging to a man or not. And depending on a woman's age or looks she can be seen as: a bird, a chick, a bit of fluff, a nice bit of stuff, a bit of skirt, a bit of crumpet, hot stuff, a doll, a bit of crackling, a gorgeous creature, an old biddy, an old bag, an old cow, or as one of us was recently called by a group of youths crossing the road near where she was standing minding her own business – a stupid old bitch! All these terms imply that women are less than human in some way, an immature or old feathered creature, an animal, a piece of fabric, a toy, a piece of meat or foodstuff. It's hard to think of similar words for adult men!

Even the apparently straightforward word 'spinster' (used to describe an unmarried woman) has a completely different attitude attached to it compared to the word 'bachelor' (used to describe an unmarried man). This is because an unmarried woman is less respected than a married woman in our society, whereas men are generally more respected no matter who they are or what they do.

So, the *words* we choose to say or write something can *also* show what we think or believe about that thing or person – even if we don't realise it at the time.

Myths and jokes about the menopause and older women, as well as about women in general, are an example of this. They are part of the social and cultural background to menopause, and can greatly affect how we feel about the menopause, and ageing.

STRESS

The effects of stress are under-estimated, and the events which may cause stress are unacknowledged, denied or trivialised. Ageism, the position of women in our society, and the way language can be used against us are all stressful. So are the more personal changes that may be taking place in our lives in middle age: the menopause, relationships changing or ending, and job or economic changes. Daily life can also be stressful: long waits for crowded buses or trains when you're exhausted and laden with bags at the end of a long day, knowing there's still more work to do when you get home.

Stress can occur in men and women of any age. It can cause flushing and sweats, palpitations of the heart, anxiety, depression, headache, indigestion, migraine, tense aching muscles, sleeplessness. It is thought that stress causes or leads to high blood pressure, angina or heart disease, ulcers and accidents.

As we saw in Chapter 1, some of the effects of stress, particularly flushing and sweats, and palpitations, are the same as those related to the fluctuating hormone levels during menopause. Menopause is often blamed for symptoms that may be caused by stress.

THE MEDICAL PROFESSION AND WOMEN'S HEALTH

One of the main sources of information about the menopause is still the medical profession. Family doctors in their surgeries, and specialists in hospitals and clinics, all voice their opinions and knowledge on the menopause to their women patients, and in the many books and articles they write on the subject. Medicine is powerful in this respect and strongly affects what people believe about the menopause.

This section looks briefly at the history and practice of medicine and its relationship to women.

Throughout the development and growth of medicine in the fifteenth and sixteenth centuries, women were systematically forced out, often being labelled as witches if they practised healing. From the middle of the sixteenth century midwives were licensed only after an appearance before a Bishop. They had to pay a fee and swear an oath that they were of good character and experienced in midwifery. The Medical Act of 1521 listed the kinds of people considered to be unsuitable to practise medicine, and included 'Smiths, Weavers and women'. Women healers were seen as dangerous amateurs whilst men developed healing and medicine as a profession, leading to the creation by the nineteenth century of a whole range of specialisms. Ironically, as women were increasingly excluded from practising medicine, their bodies became a focus for medical research and the growth of the specialism of gynaecology. As gynaecology developed, experimental surgery was performed which included removal of the clitoris, ovaries and womb – sometimes on middle-class women to 'treat' sexual desire because it was considered abnormal for these women to have such feelings.

Menopause, like other aspects of the reproductive cycles of women (e.g. pregnancy and menstruation), has been transformed by doctors from a natural event to a condition requiring medical treatment. Opinion expressed in the latter part of the nineteenth century said that sexual intercourse during or after the menopause was a 'morbid impulse' which led to haemorrhaging, tumours of the ovaries or insanity – and that it was wise for a woman to get the advice of a doctor before she married at this time in her life!

After several centuries of being excluded from the practice of medicine, women began an intense struggle in the nineteenth century to reinstate their position. Elizabeth Blackwell and Elizabeth Garrett were the first British women registered as doctors to practise, and laid the foundations for other women to study medicine. Florence Nightingale's efforts to establish nursing as a creditable profession for women also met with opposition from the medical world. Finally, during the 1870s a women's medical school was set up and clinical tuition for women students was provided by the Royal Free medical school. Today medical schools are said to be accepting about 50 per cent of women in their intake.

In medical schools women are under pressure to conform to male-orientated traditional teaching. Those who are qualified in medicine and working in the NHS are not necessarily any more concerned about the needs of women patients than their male colleagues. Also, they are unrepresentative of women from some ethnic minority groups.

A relatively small number of women manage to overcome the obstacles which prevent them from becoming consultants or specialists – the highest paid and most powerful doctors in the NHS. Whilst women form about 90 per cent of the nurses, mid-wives and lower-paid ancillary staff in hospitals, a survey in 1977 showed that only about 18 per cent of hospital doctors and 9 per cent of consultants are women, and 15 per cent of family doctors (GPs) are women. In the home women make up the majority of the large numbers of unpaid health workers. As can be seen many women are employed in medicine, but a relatively small percentage at present are in a position to change practices and policies significantly. If they do, they are likely to meet the opposition of a male-dominated administration as well as their medical colleagues.

Specialists have a *very* narrow experience of menopause because they see only a *very* small percentage of menopausal women. These are usually women who have more severe problems and have been referred to specialists by their GPs. Because specialists are regarded as the 'experts', most of us, including doctors, get our knowledge and information on the menopause from specialists: it is specialists who provide much of the available printed information. Their narrow view of menopause is reflected in their articles, books and pamphlets, so they are not really writing for the majority of women: and many women can feel quite anxious or worried after reading their information, wondering if they too will suffer from the conditions written about.

In large teaching hospitals, where most medical research takes place, it is the consultant who directs the way research funds are spent. They frequently need to try to raise funds from other sources than the Government and some of their research budget may come from the drug industry. This gives the drug companies a vested interest in the research carried out, and influences the priorities which are chosen. The menopause is of particular interest to drug companies because of the potential for the use of hormone replacement therapy (HRT) in a very large number of the female population.

In addition, the consultants can 'create' new menopause symptoms. For example, the disease of osteoporosis (which means brittle bones, and should not be confused with osteoarthritis), which can occur in a wide range of people of all ages and both sexes, is being increasingly linked to the menopause. This is part of a campaign by some specialists and drug companies to get *all* menopausal women to take hormone replacement therapy (HRT) as a preventive measure, even though 75–80 per cent of women will never develop osteoporosis.

The medical profession and the drug companies are also closely involved with the body set up to control testing and safe use of drugs – that is the Committee on the Safety of Medicines. The majority of members of the CSM and its various sub-committees are medical practitioners or pharmacists.

Since the 1960s the medical profession, which is mainly male and middle class, has been under increasing pressure from the Women's Health Movement which has criticised treatment of female patients. The formation of women's health groups and the publication of books like *Our Bodies Ourselves* have made many women more aware of the way the body functions. Increasing knowledge has helped women to challenge and question treatment and attitudes during the processes of pregnancy, childbirth and abortion. This book is part of the same questioning and challenging of attitudes and treatment.

As with pregnancy, childbirth, contraception and mental health, the menopause has now become part of medical science, which is administered, directed and controlled largely by men. Most individual women are not in any position to argue with the decisions about research carried out on our behalf, but in the past twenty years the issues have been discussed more in the open, as women joined together to demand that the medical profession take into account the needs of women as women themselves see them to be.

4 · WHAT IS THE CHANGE OF LIFE?

We have already described in Chapter 1 the changes which the menopause brings about in our bodies. In this chapter we want to think about some of the other changes which are taking place in our lives around middle age. These changes have nothing to do with the menopause, but are sometimes confused with it.

It is possible to gain a whole new lease of life in middle age, with new reserves of energy and optimism. However, many of us also go through periods of depression, emotional upset, or irritability. These feelings are often put down to the menopause itself. It is true that fluctuating hormone levels may upset our emotions, but there are often other reasons, concerned with what is happening in our day-to-day lives, which may be making us feel upset or depressed.

Such feelings are often not taken seriously by those around us. When we hear remarks like 'What do you expect at your age?' or 'It's your age, dear', it is easy to be persuaded that we have to put up with whatever is wrong, and that there is nothing we can do about it.

We believe that it is important to understand what is causing us to feel as we do (it may be one of a number of things) and take steps to do something if we are not feeling very satisfied about the way things are.

CHANGE OF ROLE

In the eyes of society, the young fertile woman plays an important role. Sexual attractiveness and being a mother are highly valued, and often regarded as signs of success and fulfilment. In recent years many women in Western countries have come to resent living by these values, and have demanded more choice about the sort of lives they lead.

However, attitudes about women die hard, and none of us can

entirely escape being affected by them. This is particularly true when we reach the menopause. It is hard to ignore the numerous unthinking comments which are directed at middle-aged women, such as 'past it' or 'old bag'. Even the word 'menopausal' can be used in a derogatory sense: for example, a woman who is justifiably angry about something can be dismissed as 'menopausal' instead of being taken seriously.

So common are such attitudes that it is not surprising that some women feel redundant and useless when they reach middle age. In reality, women in mid-life, with a third of their lives on average ahead of them after the menopause, represent a group of mature and experienced people who have a lot to contribute to society.

This is of course recognised in some other societies in which women are given greater respect as they grow older. Despite the lack of respect for middle-aged women in our society, it is still possible for mid-life to become a new opportunity for personal development, or achievement, if we want it to be (see Chapter 5).

FAMILY RELATIONSHIPS

For those women who have had children, other major changes are taking place around the time of the menopause. Children are becoming more independent: they may already have left home, got married or had a child of their own. Most of us regard these events with mixed feelings. Some of us will feel a sense of pride in our children's achievements, but there may also be feelings of loss or regret, and perhaps failure, if our children are not living up to our expectations, or have lost touch with us. We may also feel envious, or anxious that they are starting out as young adults at a time when we may feel that our own opportunities are closing in. If the children are still with us, there may be stress arising from difficult relationships. At this stage we may be delighted to find that there is now more time for ourselves; but also we may feel a sense of panic and emptiness as the children come to need us less, and we are thrown back on ourselves. Feelings such as 'What next?', 'What shall I do with the rest of my life?', 'Is this all there is?' are not uncommon, and for many of us who are mothers our relationship with our children is the closest, most affectionate one we have in our lives, so we can feel very lost and lonely when they leave home.

These events may be happening at the same time as the ending of our periods. When this happens, there may be a sense of relief for those in a sexual relationship with a man that there is no further need once the menopause is completed (see page 14) to use contraceptives. Some women are positively delighted when the menopause occurs and the monthly menstruation is over and done with. On the other hand, whether or not we have given birth to children, there is a sense of finality, that our childbearing years are now over. Those of us who wanted children, but were not able to have them, are likely to feel this more acutely. Even if we do not want more children, or have never wanted any, we may feel a sense of regret at the ending of a phase of our life to which we can never return.

Women who live in two-parent families may find that, as the children become less time-consuming, there is more energy and time left to devote to their partner. Some couples find that their relationship improves as they have more time to relax together; others reach crisis point when they are left alone with each other again. Difficulties which have been avoided can no longer be ignored, or there may be a gradual awareness between a couple that they now have little to hold them together. Middle age is often a time when men seek reassurance about their masculinity in relationships with younger women. This can be a shattering blow to a partner, and is something many women fear. A middle-aged man may appear to have plenty of choice of partners, but a middle-aged woman who loses her partner may feel a lack of confidence in her own attractiveness, because of the ways in which women of this age group are regarded.

Those of us who have a stable partner will find it helpful to involve him or her in how we are feeling about the menopause. Some women complain that male partners have little sympathy for them during the menopause. The only way men are likely to improve their knowledge and understanding is if we educate them and share with them what is happening to us.

Women partners are likely to be more understanding because both have experience of menstruation, so it is potentially easier to share feelings about the menopause with another woman.

For those of us experiencing problems in our personal relationships during mid-life, now is a good time to work on them. A useful book is *A Woman in Your Own Right* (see p.102), and Marriage

34

Guidance Councils, even for those who are not married, are usually a good source of help with difficult relationships of any kind.

CARING FOR AGED RELATIVES

In our middle years ageing relatives are likely to become more in need of support. It is usually assumed that women, rather than men, will care for elderly relatives (and even in-laws), regardless of their other responsibilities. Whilst most women are happy to offer some help to ageing relatives, that willingness is abused by 'community care' policies. They take women's caring role in the home for granted, and provide little practical or financial assistance. Caring for a frail relative can impose intolerable demands on carers, and often results in a neglect of the carer's own needs through sheer exhaustion. This is particularly true of single women, who may have the elderly relative living with them, and may not have support from a partner. A single woman is both breadwinner and carer, the usual double demand on women but without the possibility of an occasional day off. Personal life and work suffer, and, unlike caring for infants, the carer is usually more isolated and lacking support of family or social services. She may even be made to feel that it is her duty to give up paid work to care for a relative. Caring for an elderly person may also be a depressing reminder of what may be in store for the carer herself. The address of the Association of Carers is given on p.114, and it is worth enquiring locally whether there are support groups for carers in your area.

DEATH

For most of us middle age is the first time we face the death of someone close to us. Death of a close relative or friend is likely to arouse strong feelings, such as anger, guilt or depression, which are sometimes difficult to handle in a society which is embarrassed by them, and allows us little time or opportunity to mourn. Organisations which may be able to provide support at times of bereavement are listed on p.106.

EMPLOYMENT

Changes often take place in relation to paid work in mid-life. The woman who has not had a job whilst bringing up children may want to take up paid employment again; the woman who has worked part-time may be interested in increasing her hours or taking on a more responsible job. The woman who has always worked may be reassessing what she wants to do for the rest of her working life. Mid-life may also be a time to pause and reflect or to take a break from paid employment. These changes bring new excitements and achievements, but unemployment, some employers' attitudes to older women, or our own lack of self-confidence, may lead to disappointments, feelings of rejection and lack of self-worth.

APPEARANCE

The most noticeable signs of ageing – wrinkles, changing hair colour and physical limitations – not only feed into our fears about old age but also affect our feelings about ourselves and other people's responses to us.

We feel the same inside, perhaps, but we begin to look different – can that middle-aged woman I just caught sight of in a shop window really be a reflection of myself? Surely I don't really look as old as that?

We find that looks no longer attract attention or gain approval: even if we hated wolf whistles when we were younger, we notice when we do not attract them any more! We are also likely to be aware that we are no longer as 'with it' as we may have felt when we were younger, and sense that our values and opinions are different from those of younger people, and that we lack their respect because we no longer conform (if we ever did) to media images of women.

These changes sometimes have the effect of making us confused about who we are, how we should behave and how we should dress, and self-conscious about how we look. It is easy to feel that, as we are no longer young, we can no longer be attractive.

Women react in a number of different ways to changing appearance. Some try hard to conform to the television and women's magazine stereotype that we must look young to be attractive. This may involve spending a great deal of time and money on appearance, even to the extent of having face-lifts or body surgery in order to look younger. Occasionally this works for a time, but it may create an intolerable pressure to 'deliver the goods'. One of the most horrible descriptions of women who try to continue to look young is 'mutton dressed as lamb': unfortunately the fear of this phrase is enough to prevent many women from pleasing themselves about what they want to wear. As a result, the most popular solution to changing appearance is to dress in neutral or matronly clothes which are sometimes thought to be 'suitable' for middle-aged women. These have the effect of allowing the woman to fade from view, and attract as little attention as possible because she looks like a lot of other people in her age group. Even if we do not want to fade into middle age, we may have difficulty in avoiding this image as more fashionable clothes and shops are almost always designed with young women in mind. Many shops do not stock clothes in sizes over 14, and communal changing rooms can be a nightmare for anyone but the young and slim! A few chain stores are beginning to realise at last that women over 30 may still be interested in smart or more colourful, stylish clothes, but it may be too much to expect that retailers will ever think to include the over 40s or over size 14s!

Some women begin to feel in mid-life a new sense of confidence in themselves as people. If we have positive feelings about ourselves, we are likely to be less concerned about how we look to other people, and more interested in dressing in whatever gives *us* pleasure. We can wear clothes designed for younger women if that is what we want to do, and reject all those advertisements about hiding wrinkles and fighting flab for the commercial con they are.

For women who do not feel a sense of confidence in themselves, it is possible to work towards it. We hope that some of the ideas put forward in this book will help.

POSITIVE CHANGE

Whatever our individual situation, we cannot escape from the fact that the middle years bring changes for all of us. We may not like the feelings of insecurity and anxiety which change often brings, but we may also feel a sense of excitement and expectancy.

What comes out of change is partly a matter of how we react to it, and whether we are alive to new opportunities which present themselves. In middle age we have a choice between continuing to regret what we have left behind, or taking advantage of opportunities to do new and different things with our lives. It is easy to spend a lot of energy trying to pretend that things are the same, carrying on as before, trying to resist the changing patterns of our lives. The alternative is to welcome the opportunity for change, and put our energies into deciding how we would like our lives to be in the next phase. Change can lead to the opening up of new possibilities, the discovery of new aspects of ourselves. For some of us, it is a chance for which we have waited for a long time. Up to now many of us may have felt that we had little choice or control over the way our lives went; we may have allowed others to take decisions for us or just waited to see what would happen.

In the early part of adult life most women spend a lot of time looking after other people – children, partner, other relatives, bosses. In middle life it is our turn to start looking after ourselves and to make our own choices about how we want to spend our time. Women have a wide range of reactions to this realisation, from panic about how to fill the time to excitement about all the possibilities.

5 · TAKING CARE OF OURSELVES

By the time many of us reach our middle years, we have not looked after ourselves as well as we should have done. Our time and physical and emotional energy has been spent on behalf of other people, which can sometimes leave us feeling tired, fed up or depressed. The middle years can be very stressful, because of the various personal or domestic changes that may be occurring alongside the menopause. Many women say they feel they have nothing to look forward to, and dread getting older.

RECOGNISING OUR NEEDS

Men are not taught and are not expected to provide caring for women and children in the same way as women are taught to provide it for men and children. Most women are trained from early years to take care of others – starting at home with dolls. This attitude is intensified in primary, and then secondary school, where housecraft or domestic science still tends to be taken by girls, and woodwork, metalwork and electronics, etc, by boys. Efforts are being made by some local education authorities to alter this practice because it reinforces the traditional male and female roles, and these can be the source of domestic conflict in families in adult life.

Many girls drop their sporting and physical leisure activities when they reach adolescence, even if they were lucky enough to go to a school that encouraged them in the first place! At this age there is great pressure on young women to stop being 'tomboys' and to concentrate on being attractive to boys. This all too often entails dieting – which can interfere with the hormone system and prevent menstruation and ovulation, and learning 'how to please or serve others', instead of themselves. Popular culture such as songs, magazines, comics, television and films all urge women to be 'good to their men' and give them what they need. This and the fact that men are not expected to possess domestic skills ensures that everyone comes to accept women's role as the carers: responsible for the physical and emotional health and needs of others.

But nowhere along the line are we as women taught or encouraged to recognise our own real emotional, physical and psychological needs.

Whether we are aiming for a more satisfying job or career, or want to take up sports, hobbies or leisure pursuits, the needs of the family or others are always seen as coming first. We are often thought of as selfish – and can actually *feel* selfish – if we consider ourselves and want to go out, leaving the family/dependants to look after themselves. If we complain, we are seen as 'women's libbers', or nagging women.

It is not at all selfish to look after ourselves and our health, particularly around the menopause. In fact it is very important that we do so, because no-one else is likely to. The more we understand the needs of our bodies and look after ourselves before and during the menopause, the more likely we are to be able to deal with problems, should they arise.

OSTEOPOROSIS (POROUS OR BRITTLE BONES)

It is very important to encourage all young women to take more care of themselves, and develop a life-style which includes the right diet and exercise, in a way which will build up their bones to be strong enough to resist the effects of the increased bone loss which seems to occur after menopause. This would reduce the 20–25 per cent of women over 70 who end up in hospital with serious fractures which will not mend.

In any case, for women, a routine of good diet and exercise, which should have been a habit since youth, becomes *crucial* by middle age, in order to resist the increased bone loss after menopause. Medical evidence suggests that this is more critical in slim white women and all women who smoke, while black women of African descent seem to experience less bone loss, have stronger bones to start with, and get less osteoporosis in older age.

Anyone is likely to get osteoporosis if they are sedentary and not getting the right form of exercise. For instance, astronauts suffer from calcium loss from the bones as a result of being weightless in space. This has been compared to anyone (young or old, male or female) lying immobile in hospital for any length of time, where the same problem occurs. *Unused bones lose calcium.* The bones become more and more porous, and eventually, if calcium loss continues over a period of years, it develops into osteoporosis and the bones begin to fracture and crumble.

Exercise against the force of gravity, such as brisk walking, dancing, skipping, jogging and games like tennis, badminton and football, will all help to prevent calcium leaking from the bones, and can reverse the situation – making bones stronger.

From childhood, the bones of both sexes are being built up (depending on exercise and adequate diet). Then after age 30–35 both sexes gradually begin to lose bone (again depending on life-style and diet). Some women have less dense bones than men, and seem to lose bone at a slightly faster rate than men. This may be because many women have a less or differently active life-style to men, or because many women do not nourish themselves properly when they are younger. Perhaps because they feed everyone else in the family first and eat what's left over, or because they are often dieting. It is also related to inadequate exposure to sunlight, or to genetic, or hormonal factors.

EXERCISE AND RELAXATION

Exercise and relaxation can become really essential for our well-being in mid-life. We are entitled to spend time and energy on ourselves to get some *personal* pleasure and enjoyment out of life. This will help us to value ourselves as people more, and help to prevent us becoming depressed as we cope with the daily stresses in our lives. Equally important, exercise will keep our bodies (muscles, bones, sinews, lungs, heart, circulation, organs, digestion etc) in good shape and delay the ageing process. Ageing depends on diet, and the use, disuse, misuse or abuse we subject our bodies to. Smoking, bad eating habits or diet, sedentary or heavy jobs, can all either misuse or abuse our bodies. If we do not start to nourish and exercise them properly to counteract this then our bodies will age more quickly, and we can also become more prone to gynaecological and menopausal problems.

Taking care of ourselves can also be an enjoyable and very sociable experience. Because most of us are very busy and often feel tired a lot of the time, the idea of exercise at home can seem pretty dull – and it takes a lot of self-discipline to do it by ourselves!

By far the best idea is to join a keep-fit, exercise, dance or movement class at the local school, community centre or college, with a friend or by ourselves. This means that we can have regular outings of our *own* each week, away from jobs, chores and responsibilities. We will meet people and have fun. And, of course, we will be getting the exercise that will keep our bodies in good working order, and help us to relax and *feel* good.

N.B. Before starting on strenuous exercise of any sort, you should have a check-up with your doctor.

DANCE

Dance can be a very pleasurable way of getting the sort of exercise which will strengthen our bones, whilst keeping us fit. There are some good classes around where older women can feel comfortable, particularly those run by the Keep Fit Association or local Adult Education Institutes, etc.

During the dance-exercise boom in the early 1980s, great emphasis was placed on the young slim-sexy fashion-conscious body. The craze had much more to do with *looking* good for the effect it had on members of the opposite sex, rather than *feeling* good and healthy for sheer personal fun and enjoyment, regardless of what shape we are.

The craze put a lot of older women off or made us feel shy about joining classes because we were embarrassed about our bodies.

The majority of women going to Keep Fit Association classes are over 30, so don't be put off or give up looking for a class where you will feel relaxed and have fun!

YOGA

Many women find yoga a restful and calming way of staying fit and healthy. Again, check with your local school, community centre or college for classes, and find one that you can really enjoy. There are a number of different kinds of yoga, and if you want to find out which sort will suit you best it is possible to attend Adult Education Institutes as a *visitor*. This arrangement exists to enable people to make the right choice before committing themselves. The benefits of yoga are physical and mental, and you do as much or as little as you want. *No-one* need feel she's not fit enough to join a yoga class.

SWIMMING

Women who learn to swim for the first time in middle age or later years are frequently delighted to find something which gives them so much pleasure. It's often possible to find a pool nearby but it is best to check to see if they have a women-only or adults-only session, and go then. Otherwise, avoid the children's rush hour so that you can feel relaxed. Anyone who chooses swimming should also make sure she walks a lot, or does some other exercise as well. Although swimming is the finest source of exercise for muscles and internal organs, it doesn't exercise bones. Because we are weightless in water – like the astronauts in space – swimming won't prevent bone loss.

WALKING

One of the most under-rated forms of exercise for strengthening our bones is walking. This doesn't mean a quick dash to the shops or launderette and back, loaded down with bags, but an hour, or even half an hour, 2 to 3 times a week. If you can't manage this, anything is better than nothing – walk as much as you can, as often as you can. When you walk, really stride out. Relax your shoulders, and breathe deeply as you look around and notice things you have never seen before because you are usually thinking of what you've got to do next! Whether it's around local familiar streets, or a nearby park, or out in the country, giving yourself the space, time and freedom to enjoy what you see around you as you walk can be a new and liberating experience. But walk briskly. Don't stroll or saunter!

Medical evidence suggests that 2–3 good brisk walks per week can slow down or stop bone loss. Sufficient vigorous walking might reverse the process and strengthen bone.

OTHER FORMS OF EXERCISE

If you feel you would like to take up some other sport or physical activity (like jogging, or gymnasium activities, or joining a walking or rambling club, among many, many others) contact your local Health Education Unit, your local Adult Education Institute, or write to the Sports Education Council (address on p.113) for their package of leaflets with suggested ideas and contacts for the over-40 age group.

RELAXATION EXERCISES

Doing any form of physical exercise will help us to relax. Yoga is particularly good. But there are specific exercises if we feel very tense and anxious, under pressure or stress. It's a good idea to check with the local health centre or health education worker to see if they have got a relaxation/stress group or class set up. If not, write to 'Relaxation for Living' (see p.109) for their leaflet on how to breathe properly to relax.

Most of us use only a small proportion of our lungs and breathe far too shallowly: this can reduce our circulation and be the cause of dizziness, tiredness, palpitations, anxiety etc. Try lying on your back flat on the floor; tightening and then relaxing each limb and part of the body in turn, starting with your toes and working up to the top of your head; empty your mind; breathe regularly and deeply for about 10–15 minutes.

Start gradually, as the sudden increase in oxygen when you aren't used to it can also make you feel faint! Do this in the evenings before you go to bed if you can find a quiet, uninterrupted space – or whenever you can.

KEGEL EXERCISES

These were originally developed as post-natal exercises, but *all* women should *in any case* practise these exercises daily, as a matter of course, to keep the pelvic region in good firm elastic shape, and to help prevent any problems occurring in the future.

If you have got gynaecological/pelvic aches and pains or symptoms, say stress incontinence (leaking drops of urine if you laugh, cough or sneeze), prolapse, or a dry or sore vagina, these are exercises which will help you. They are fully described on p. 99.

DIET

We are often told that we get all the minerals and vitamins we need from our normal daily diet. But much food today is either highly processed, or stale by the time we get it. Cooking reduces even further the vitamins and minerals that remain. Also, for many of us, canteen or convenience food is a large part of our diet which limits the range of fresh or wholesome food we actually eat in a week. This means that some of us may need to take vitamins or minerals in tablet form to supplement our dietary intake.

Diet is important because we need to help our bones resist the increased calcium loss in the years immediately after menopause. Recommendations from nutritional and bone specialists say that from about the age of 30–35 women require in the region of 700–1000 mg of calcium per day. The daily requirement increases to 1000–1500 mg per day after the age of 45, or after the menopause. Vitamin D is also required to help the body absorb calcium properly.

It is unlikely that many of us get the total amount of calcium we need from our daily diet unless we are in the habit of drinking nearly 2 pints of milk a day! (Skimmed milk is very good by the way because it has very low fat content, but has a higher calcium level than ordinary full or half cream milk, so one pint gives 761 mg.) Sesame seeds or tahini are very calcium-rich, as are sardines or pilchards (because you eat the bones too). Also dark greens like watercress, spring greens or kale are calcium-rich. If you still think you need to supplement your diet, get a bottle of calcium tablets from your chemist or health food shop – but notice that they come in different forms and strengths. Some people feel that calcium is easier for the body to use if taken in the form of bonemeal tablets, or dolomite – which is a combination of calcium and magnesium – another important mineral.

The main dietary sources of Vitamin D are oily fish (mackerel, herring, salmon, tuna, sardines etc) egg yolk, and butter. Soft margarine-type spreads and some cereals have Vitamin D added to them during manufacture, so many of us probably get sufficient Vitamin D if we eat these foods. We also get Vitamin D from the exposure of our skin to sunlight. If we have had a hot summer, or been to a sunny climate for a holiday, the body will store Vitamin D for some weeks afterwards.

N.B. Vitamin D supplements should be taken *very* cautiously, if at all, as too much is dangerous. Only very elderly people usually need some Vitamin D supplement.

We also need a healthy diet to nourish our nervous and circulatory systems, and keep our sinews, muscles and internal organs in good shape. Alcohol, smoking and medicines like antibiotics, oral contraceptives or hormone replacement (HRT) can play havoc with the hormone and digestive systems, greatly increasing our need for Vitamins such as B complex, and E. Vitamin C, contained in fresh citrus fruit, is needed *daily* to help the body utilise all the other vitamins and minerals effectively: it can be supplied by, say, an orange a day.

RELATIONSHIPS: SHARING, AND GROUPS

Because many of us spend a large part of our lives looking after others, with little time or encouragement to go out and socialise on our own or with other women, and because very few of us retain our friendships with women after we leave school, we can often find ourselves feeling isolated and lonely as we get older. Marriages or relationships may end through death or separation, children leave home, older or sick relatives may need more, or full-time, caring. Just at the time of life when many of us need the affectionate support and friendship of a 'best friend' or a circle or group of good close women friends, we may find we have no-one we can really talk to or go and do things with. More and more women are starting to go to an evening or day class or club at a local college or centre. They are joining women's groups – perhaps a menopause/mid-life group, or a health group, or an assertiveness training group, and are finding a whole new lease of life as a result: friends, a good laugh, and something interesting to do. Learning more about ourselves gives us self-assurance and confidence.

Having good women friends to share things with is important for all of us: once we've taken the first perhaps rather scary step ourselves by making the first move to go to a class, club or group, the rest becomes much easier. Even if we don't make good friends on that first occasion, it will give us the confidence to try another group or class.

Most women outlive men, and the people we are really going to need later in life are our close women friends. There are millions of elderly women living by themselves all over the country, often feeling lonely and isolated, when they could be socialising together, and supporting each other in a happier and more enjoyable way.

SEXUALITY

Sexuality can be a joy or a problem, or not a very important part of our lives, which we may feel happy or unhappy about. Unfortunately, for many people, sexuality and having sex have come to mean the same thing. Sex has become divorced from sensuality, particularly within traditional couple relationships in our society.

Our sensual feelings are, literally, our feelings in response to our senses being stimulated: touching ourselves, things or other people, being touched, stroked by skin on skin, hands, feet, tongues, noses, ears, or pleasing fabrics. 'I love the feel of clean fresh sheets after a hot bath', as one of us said when writing this book. There are also visual experiences, or smells, or warmth, coolness, sounds, eating or drinking enjoyable things. All of these and much more are sensual experiences, or can be. Our sensuality is part of our sexuality and sexuality is part of our sensuality. We can experience them with other people or by ourselves.

Unfortunately, many sexual relationships either lose their sensuality over the course of time, or sensuality may never have been a feature. Some women find this very frustrating, especially in relationships with those men who just want to get quick physical satisfaction. This attitude denies the existence of a woman's sexual feelings except as a response to his. It also ignores the existence of sensuality for both of them: those delicious sensual feelings that can occur from touch all over the body if they are not simply focussed on rapid orgasm (usually his) as the one and only form of sex. Hours of pleasure and excitement can be had with never an orgasm occurring!

There are many conflicting messages to do with good or bad women in our society, concerning sexuality and women's sexual behaviour. All too often, as women, we are inhibited about touching our own bodies. We may have been taught to believe that masturbation is wrong, or, worse still, dirty in some way. Or that only bad women really enjoy sexual feelings. This means that we know very little about our own bodies and our own sexuality: the different things that feel enjoyable to us, what we enjoy doing or having done to us. But if we feel free to explore our own bodies and learn to be loving to ourselves, we discover more fully our own sexuality. We can learn to look after and take 'care' of ourselves sexually in a pleasurable way if we feel we need or want to, whether we are in relationships with others, or by ourselves from choice or circumstances. Masturbation also helps to keep the pelvic area in a healthy condition, and can increase vaginal moistness.

For women who are celibate from choice, or because of circumstances, masturbation or self-pleasuring can be a comfortable, enjoyable and guilt-free option. Some women in heterosexual relationships find that, after menopause, they enjoy sex far more than before because the fear of pregnancy has gone. Other women find they go 'off' sex: perhaps they never really enjoyed it very much and felt sex was over-rated. Possibly their partner always expects penetration, and is unwilling or uninterested in trying more sensitive or sensual forms of love-making that allow a woman to become sufficiently aroused – this directly affects the amount of moisture produced by the vagina. Dryness of the vagina is then blamed on the menopause, when in fact it may be due to low arousal and desire. Tiredness, or a dry or tender vagina, can become the reasons for loss of sexual interest (even though they needn't be), because the real reasons may seem too difficult to solve. Many women feel unable to talk to their partner about their sexual activity, perhaps wanting to suggest different ways of making love but unable to speak about it. It's easier to blame the menopause, and leave it at that, than to get into a situation that might lead to rows and misunderstandings – which may well happen in such a sensitive matter if a couple have not previously been in the habit of talking to each other about their sex life and love-making. Some women find that masturbation becomes a much more enjoyable form of sexual activity: you can please yourself and there are no arguments!

For women in relationships with women, any difficulties in communicating about sexual problems or needs are potentially made easier by a closer understanding of each other's bodies and sexual geography. Menstruation is nearly always an experience in common: the menopause is, or will be, another common experience. If there are reasons for wanting to change or vary love-making or sexual activities, it may be possible to discuss and understand them more readily and easily.

RELATIONSHIP COUNSELLING

If you are in a relationship of any sort that is a problem you could seek help from a marriage guidance counsellor. Although the name might put some people off because it sounds as though it's only for married people, they are experienced in helping with *any* stressful or unhappy relationship whether heterosexual, lesbian, married or unmarried, and also parent/child relationships, i.e. you and a son or daughter, or you and a parent. There are also many other agencies and groups to turn to if you would like help or advice, or just someone to talk to about a particular problem – if you have a sick or elderly dependant and no-one to help or support you, for example. In addition, disabled people are involved in running their own organisations to offer support and help of various kinds.

It is sometimes possible to bring change into unsatisfactory sexual relationships if we are prepared to work on them. Some excellent books have been written, which give helpful advice on improving sexual relationships, and these are listed on p.113.

6 · MAKING THE CHANGES WE WANT

It is essential that we get to know and acknowledge ourselves as whole people. Just as we are not encouraged to get to know and understand our bodies, the same is true about getting to know our emotional needs.

Most of us have achieved nothing like our full potential by the time we reach the menopause. We have held back and denied so much in the interest of 'femininity', or being a 'good' wife or mother, or both. Now is the time when we can reclaim some of the lost parts of ourselves; skills and interests which we gave up or did not pursue when we were younger; qualities which were not compatible with our previous life-style, or which we were told were 'unladylike' or unacceptable for other reasons.

REASSESSING OUR LIVES

What are we going to do during the next phase of our lives? How do we want to be? What do we want to achieve? These are very difficult questions for women because we are not used to planning or being responsible for our own lives. We tend to believe that we have no control over what happens. We usually just wait and see. We leave the planning to other people – parents, husbands, family etc. Many of us are still carrying round the 'dos and don'ts', 'shoulds and shouldn'ts', from our childhood, and these enormously restrict our adult lives. Whenever we say out loud or to ourselves I should ... I must ... I shouldn't ... I mustn't ... it's a good idea to try to identify who is really saying this, or where we got these ideas from. Is it really me, or is it something that was said to me when I was a little girl? If so, is it really something I want to continue with? Try saying out loud '*I* am now in charge of my life, and *I* will decide what I am going to do'.

GETTING STARTED

Getting to know ourselves is the first step towards reassessing our lives, and it is a good idea to begin by looking back over what has happened so far. There are several ways to do this. You will get much more out of this section if you can share your thinking with a friend, or do the exercises together and compare notes.

One idea is to write about ourselves and our lives, a kind of autobiography for no-one to read but ourselves; or a diary describing our moods and feelings as they change through the days and weeks. Some women keep a diary of their menopause or their menstrual cycle, noting down all the changes they notice in their bodies and moods, and looking for patterns during the cycle. Start trying to recognise and understand your own feelings, both physical and emotional.

Another way of thinking about your life so far is to complete a mid-life questionnaire. You will find an example of this in Appendix 3.

Alternatively, you could make a drawing or chart of your life so far. Depict in any way you like the most important events of your life, starting from birth, or earlier if you know anything about what happened to your parents before you were born which might have affected your life. Put in the people who influenced your life, the ups and downs, births, relationships, deaths, successes and failures, the decisions, the turning points. Leave plenty of space because you will keep thinking of things you have left out. When you have finished, try to understand the patterns and themes of your life. For instance, how did you deal with the disappointments? Is there a pattern? Do you give in easily? Get angry? Take on challenges? What kind of person are you?

Following on from this, try another exercise. Write down all the things you are good at. Most women find this very difficult. We tend to underestimate and devalue our skills. We are much better at recognising what we're not good at. But, if we stop and think, we will begin to realise what a staggering number of skills it takes to run a house or flat, bring up children, manage a family budget, organise a babysitting group, nurse or look after sick or injured members of the family, hold down a job, often at the same time as all these other things. Many of the skills we use on a daily basis, such as being a good listener, planning and cooking a meal or organising a family's activities, are just not recognised or valued. To list all our skills can help to increase our confidence, and may give ideas about what to do. If you find it difficult to write down what you are good at, keep a list over a week of all the things you enjoy doing (these are some of the things you are likely to be good at). Ask your family and friends what they think you are good at. It is possible for *every* woman reading this to come up with a long list of skills.

Here are two exercises which may help you to think about the future. Sit back in a comfortable chair, close your eyes, relax and daydream about the future. If you had an entirely free hand, if you could do anything you wanted, what would your life be like? Follow your imagination, give full rein to it, picture where you would live, who would live with you, how you would spend your time. When you have finished, write down in as much detail as you can what came into your mind.

Sit back and close your eyes again. Then project yourself forward in time to when you are very old. How would you like people to remember you as you were in middle-life, how would you like to have been, what would you have liked to achieve?

Although these are fantasies, they may give you ideas about what you could do in the here and now, what kind of person you would like to be, or what you would like to be doing.

Exercises like these are often used in Life Planning Workshops. They might have titles like 'Assessing ourselves' or 'Where next?' Keep a watch to see if there are any being held in your Adult Education Institute or local college.

The Open University course 'Work Choices' in the Community Education series is another way of following up on some of these ideas at home. Such exercises are designed to help us open up our thinking about what we want to do, and what we are capable of, and are not only to do with jobs and careers.

When thinking about middle age, we usually pick on all the disadvantages. It is worth thinking what the advantages are. Exercises like the one above on listing our skills may help us to recognise some of the things which we have achieved in our lives. Many of us have more time to ourselves when we reach mid-life; we may feel we have more freedom to do what we want to do, and to say what we think (we don't care as much as we did, maybe, what other people think of us); some of us have more self-confidence; some may even have more money.

MAKING CHANGES

It may take a long time to decide exactly what it is we want for ourselves in the next phase of our lives. It's a good idea to think it out in as much detail as possible, and ideas to help you do this will be given later. Most of us will be aware of some changes we want to make, and it is important to start on these as soon as possible. Make the changes small at first. For example, decide to put aside an afternoon or evening every week to do something that you would find enjoyable for yourself. You might decide to join a yoga class, go out with a friend, or just loll around doing nothing, if that is what you would enjoy. It is better to tackle something easy first. Once you have begun it gets easier. It's a good idea to keep a note of what you are thinking and what changes you decide to make. Reading back over this will remind you of what you have done and give you encouragement as you go along.

Making changes and beginning new things is not easy. For most of us there are fears, setbacks and practical problems which block our progress.

Change often means giving up or losing something of what we have at the moment. It's hard to give up the security of the old familiar patterns. Where will these changes lead? Do I dare to take the plunge? Can I take the risk of letting go of what I have at the moment? What will other people think? Will I lose the acceptance of my friends, partner, children? Although everyone agrees that middle-aged women should be able to develop their own interests, relatives do not like having their comfortable routines upset because mum is out more often, and male partners often become uncomfortable when a woman starts getting her life together and becoming less dependent. It is a good idea to anticipate such objections, and keep friends and relatives in touch with our plans. They are less likely to object if their co-operation is sought. But do not be surprised if misunderstandings occur. A man who has believed all his life that a woman's place is in the home may find it very upsetting when his wife announces that she has other ideas. Elderly relatives may fear that they will get less attention if their daughter takes up interests of her own.

Some of the objections may even come from yourself. Most of us are very good at finding reasons for not doing things. For example: the children (or partner, or dependent relative) need me to cook the tea ... my husband won't let me ... I'm not clever enough. ... Think about the excuses or reasons you normally use. If you learn to recognise them they are less likely to work, because, although they might *seem* like good reasons, they really are not. If you truly want to do something for yourself you will find ways of dealing with all the reasons you think you have for not doing it.

Don't expect to do everything yourself. Seek help, pick other people's brains, talk to as many other women as possible. Better still, try to find a woman friend to join you.

Even if there are some setbacks and disappointments, don't give up once you have started! If 50 per cent of your attempts come off, you are doing very well. Be patient with yourself, and do not expect too much. Reward yourself when you achieve something, however small. If you start something and then find that you are not enjoying it, don't feel you *have* to carry on – just please yourself. Allow yourself the luxury of making some mistakes, but don't let them put you off.

The rest of this chapter is about ideas and resources for possible new directions in mid-life.

EDUCATION AND TRAINING

Many middle-aged women opt for some kind of education, either as a way of improving qualifications, or to follow a particular interest, or as a way of getting back to work. If you are not sure what to do with your time a course is always a good start, as it puts you in touch with other people and opens up opportunities.

Some women lack confidence about starting or returning to study. We fear we are out of touch, too stupid, too slow, too old. Nowadays people of *all* ages study, and many courses welcome mature women, who are often considered more stimulating to teach than younger people. Teachers on such courses have often chosen to work with adults, because they have had the experience of being a mature student themselves. Some courses are specially designed for women returners. Most young students enjoy having older colleagues and are usually happy for older women to join their social gatherings. They appreciate the sense of realism and the experience brought by older people to discussions. It is easy to imagine that learning will be more difficult for someone who has not studied for a long time – 'you can't teach an old dog new tricks'. However, many women who have returned to study in mid-life have found that age is not a barrier to learning, and that having a breadth of experience and knowledge is a great advantage. There are courses available that teach study and learning techniques for those who have never studied before, or not for a long time.

Much persistence is needed to find a way around the different courses on offer and to acquire all the relevant information, so don't be put off if it is difficult. Try following up some of the ideas listed below.

(1) If you are unsure about your real interest in studying or training or need to start at the beginning, try:

(a) A course at your local Adult Education Institute or university Extra Mural Department. Some Adult Education Institutes offer very basic courses in writing, spelling, grammar, maths, etc, for people who do not have confidence in these skills. Information is available from your local library.

(b) A special course for women 'returners'. NOW courses (New Opportunities for Women), New Horizons or Fresh Start courses are designed to help women who wish to return to work or study after a long gap, to look at options available for further study or job training. No qualifications are needed, and the fees are very low. The courses last for six weeks, and include job sampling, counselling, help with applications and interview techniques. Information is available from your local library about colleges offering such courses.

(2) If you need advice about courses which are available to you, contact:

(a) Your local library.

(b) Your local Further Education College or Adult Education Institute, either of which may have a free specialist educational advisory service for adults or educational guidance department. The Advisory Council for Adult and Continuing Education, 19b De Montford Street, Leicester LE1 7GE, also provides a list of these services.

(3) If you want to work towards a more academic course, you could consider the following:

(a) There are a small number of colleges for adults only, providing preparation courses in academic work. Details of these are listed in 'Opportunities in higher education for mature students', obtainable from CNAA, 344/354 Grays Inn Road, London WC1X 8PB.

(b) There is one college which caters for women only: Hillcroft College, South Bank, Surbiton, Surrey KT6 6DF.

(c) Polymaths and polyphysics courses are designed for older people who wish to prepare for 'A' levels or degrees (information from Institute of Maths and its Application, Maitland House, Warrior Square, Southend on Sea, Essex SS1 2JY, and Dr J. A. Shaw, Physics Group, Hatfield Polytechnic, PO Box 109, Hatfield, Herts AI10 9AB.

(d) Access courses are for people without qualifications. Information is available from your local Further Education College.

(4) If you need information about grants, write for 'Grants to Students – a Brief Guide', to D.E.S., Room 2/11, Elizabeth House, York Road, London SE1 7PH, or contact the Scottish Education Department, Awards Branch, Haymarket House, 7 Clifton Terrace, Edinburgh EH12 5DT.

(5) If you live out of reach of colleges or adult education, investigate distance learning schemes. The Open University, Walton Hall, Milton Keynes MK7 6AA, provides a wide range of courses, which can be taken on a very flexible basis. Fee reductions are available for unemployed people. Many other correspondence courses are available through the National Extension College, 10 Brookland Avenue, Cambridge CB2 2HN (see also p.109).

PAID EMPLOYMENT

There may not be any choice about returning to or continuing in paid employment. Many women applying for jobs when they are middle-aged fear that they are too old. Whilst it is true that many employers are prejudiced against older women, it is worth remembering that many others prefer older women because they have valuable life experience, and they are considered to be more reliable

56

and mature than younger people. This is a point on which to sell yourself.

(1) If you do not know what work you want to do or are seeking a change of job, try:

(a) 'Work Choices', the Open University continuing education course.
(b) Your local Further Education College or local education authority careers service.
(c) The National Advisory Service on Careers for Women, Drayton House, 30 Gordon Street, London WC1H 0AX. They offer a fee-paying advice service and literature for sale.

(2) If you lack experience or qualifications, you could:

(a) Take a WOW course (Wider Opportunities for Women). These are either full- or part-time, and are designed for women who want to obtain unskilled or semi-skilled jobs. Women who attend a WOW course are paid for attending them. Information is obtainable from your local Job Centre.
(b) Take a TOPS course (Training Opportunities Scheme). These are full-time, free and varied in length, and exist to train people for particular skills like printing, carpentry, computing and book-keeping. A weekly allowance is paid for attending them. Information is available at your local Job Centre.
(c) Do some voluntary work to gain experience (see under 'Other Possibilities' below).

SELF-EMPLOYMENT

If there are no suitable jobs in your area, it is worth considering self-employment. This requires a marketable idea, energy and commitment. There are two organisations which publish useful booklets and give advice on setting up a small business: the Small Firms Service, Freefone 2444 (England), 846 (Scotland), 1208 (Wales), and the Council for Small Industries in Rural Areas, 141 Castle Street, Salisbury, Wilts. There are also courses available (information from your local Further Education College or Small Firms Service). Some Job Centres also supply information on self-employment.

It is worth considering whether any of your practical skills can

57

be used to set yourself up in business. For example, if you enjoy cooking, sewing or knitting, you could set up a market stall (details from your Town Hall), advertise your products or run a mail-order business. In one outer London borough a group of women rent a café and run it in turns on a daily basis. Some of them then go on to run their own business. Other skills which you already possess may enable you to earn money, for example, through fostering or minding children, looking after elderly people, hairdressing or driving. Project Fullemploy, Unit 120, Clerkenwell Workshops, 31 Clerkenwell Close, London EC1R 0AT, runs a self-employment resource centre, and courses for women only in London, Bristol and Sandwell. There are lots of other ideas in a book called *Creating Your Own Work* (see p.111) which also gives advice on all aspects of self-employment.

OTHER POSSIBILITIES

For some women paid work may either seem impossible or not essential if there is another breadwinner in the house.

If you are in this situation you may decide to use the time and opportunity of mid-life to take up an interest which you have had for many years, or one you wish to develop, e.g. painting, pottery, writing, singing, photography, rambling, cycling, carpentry or weaving, to mention but a very few. There are usually a variety of classes or courses available to improve skills or widen interests. There may also be groups in your area, for example creative writing groups. Some of the many courses available are listed in *Creating Your Own Work*.

Most voluntary organisations depend on women for survival. A lot of voluntary work is thankless and exploited, but there are also opportunities for different kinds of rewarding work which can also provide useful experience or training for those who wish to go on to paid work. Consult your local Council for Voluntary Service, settlement, volunteer bureau or library for details of work available in your area. Other volunteer jobs are advertised in *New Society* or local magazines (such as *City Limits* in London). Some voluntary organisations offer training for the job, for example Citizens' Advice Bureaux, and some provide support groups.

One of the writers of this book is an example of a woman who changed course in mid-life, and is continuing to develop her interests. She left school aged 16 with a few 'O' levels. Within ten years she had married, had three children, was divorced and earning her living with whatever typing jobs she could fit in to her childcaring. When she was 35, she took a full-time secretarial job, and two years later she decided to start doing some evening classes for fun. This led to her taking a Diploma Course part-time for two years, which gave her the confidence to apply for a full time M.A. course. She was accepted even though she had no first degree. She got paid time off from her employers because the course related to her job. For her dissertation, she decided to look at ageing and the menopause and, as a result of this work and study, she then decided to design and teach courses on the menopause, to share the information with other women. Approaching the age of 50, she is now plucking up the courage to escape her secretarial job after more than 13 years, and concentrate on part-time teaching and writing to earn her living. Through the work on the menopause, she met the other two writers of this book, and we all decided to work together as much as possible. We were then approached by Blandford Press to write this book.

7 · SEEKING ADVICE AND INFORMING OURSELVES ABOUT THE MENOPAUSE

A recent television programme on the menopause resulted in a very large response from women asking for further information on the subject. From our experiences of talking to women about the menopause, we know that women want more and better information. Some women we have talked to wished that their families had been better informed too, and said that this would have helped when they had their menopause.

A number of women we talked to said that they just wanted confirmation that they were going through the menopause, and that what they were experiencing was part of a natural process. Being reassured that we are not alone in our feelings and experiences, and that our own particular worry can be shared, is very helpful.

If we have reliable information, we can talk to doctors more confidently, for example about the risks and advantages of hormone replacement therapy. If we know what to expect and what we can do for ourselves when we reach the menopause we can be more in control of our lives. The more we can talk about the menopause to our partners and family, the more they are likely to understand what it means for us.

FAMILY DOCTORS

Many women go at some point to their doctor for advice about the menopause. It is often not a very satisfactory experience, because the doctor is too busy. Male doctors sometimes do not seem to understand what it really feels like to be in the menopause. Generally speaking, GPs receive very little training on the menopause when they are students, and so do not know very much about it. Women consulting their GPs with hot flushes are more likely to be taken seriously, but women with depression, PMT, tiredness, or aches and pains may be dismissed. Either way, many women may be told they 'will just have to get on with it', or may be handed a prescription for sleeping pills or tranquillisers, without any real investigation into their symptoms. Sometimes symptoms of other, perhaps serious, conditions may not be checked out, and are dismissed as 'merely the menopause'. In order to take more control of the situation and get the answers you want, it helps to write down a list of questions to take to the surgery.

CLINICS AND CENTRES

Menopause clinics were set up to provide women with access to a doctor with special interest in the menopause and the time to discuss it fully. Menopause clinics are usually part of a large teaching hospital where all the consultants are involved in a research programme. Attending a clinic often means that you are part of the research. In the case of the menopause, the research frequently involves the use and safety of hormone replacement therapy, and is often funded by drug companies. A teaching hospital should have good facilities for the necessary health checks for anyone taking HRT for any length of time – especially for several months or longer (see p. 71).

Well Woman Clinics are few and far between. Again they are usually part of the NHS, but are often more relaxed and informal than surgeries or hospitals. Some voluntary organisations run Well Woman Clinics, for which a charge is made.

Sometimes the local Health Education Unit takes a particular interest in menopause and can be another source of information.

In some areas of the country there are Women's Health Groups, Menopause Groups and Women's Therapy Centres. As they are run by women, they are likely to see things from a woman's point of view. One very important Centre is the Women's Health Information Centre (see p.102). This provides information and runs workshops on any aspect of health which affects women. Questions are dealt with on the phone, and information can be sent through the post, sometimes for a small charge, but usually free (be sure to send a stamped addressed envelope!).

VALUING OUR OWN KNOWLEDGE

What women have to say for themselves from their own experience has, until recently, been the least valued of all knowledge. This is particularly the case with women from cultures other than white Western European, with the result that much available information is racist in attitude. This is changing as more women's health groups are set up, and as more women doctors and researchers become interested in the subject. For example, there are studies now taking place to find out from their own experience what the menopause means to women of different cultural backgrounds, and why some women have an easy menopause, whereas for others it is more difficult. Another question which is being asked by women researchers is what effect taking the pill for contraception might have on the menopause. Again, women's own experiences will provide the answers.

We had hoped in this book to be able to provide information which is equally relevant to women from cultural groups other than our own. Unfortunately, we have not yet been able to obtain the information we were seeking. The only group we have heard of which is exploring the menopause in relation to a variety of cultural groups is in North London.

SELF-HELP GROUPS

In the past few years, many kinds of self-help groups have been started by people who were not in the medical profession, but who wanted to share information, problems and solutions with other people like themselves. The most well-known group is probably Alcoholics Anonymous, which has been going for many years, but there are also many other groups, for example for hysterectomy, migraine and endometriosis.

A self-help group is a small informal group, which does not rely on experts to run it. It recognises that we *all* possess a lot of knowledge which is valuable to share. Most women find self-help groups very useful and great fun. They are also a very good way of meeting new friends. A self-help group meets regularly to offer its members support, encouragement and understanding, and to exchange ideas, practical suggestions and information. What happens and how it runs is up to its members to decide.

STARTING A MENOPAUSE GROUP

Anyone can start a group. You may know one or two other women who would be interested in joining, but aim for between five and nine members. There are some much bigger groups, but it is probably better to split up into small groups so that members can get to know each other.

It may be necessary to advertise to get enough women to start a group. Put up a notice in the local clinic, or community centre, Well Woman Clinic or GP's surgery. Ask your local health visitor to spread the word. You could also advertise in the local paper or *Spare Rib* magazine. When wording the advertisement, phrase it to include any woman who is interested – some women may just want to find out what others experience before they reach the menopause themselves. If you can, make it easy for enquirers to get hold of you. They may be embarrassed if a man answers the phone, so if there are men in your household, make sure everyone in the house knows about the ad. It is worth asking the local paper if they would be interested in writing an article on the menopause and including details of the new group starting. Be prepared for anything to happen. Some ads attract very few enquirers, others have been known to attract over 70.

It is a good idea to hold an open meeting in a public place before the group gets started properly, so that women can come without committing themselves. It is usually possible to get free access to rooms in community centres or clinics. The first meeting can decide where the group is going to meet when it gets going, at what time, for how long, and whether more than one group is needed. The group can either continue to meet in a public place if somewhere sufficiently comfortable and private can be found, or in group members' homes.

PLANNING THE GROUP

If the group decides to meet in members' homes, it is better not to meet at the same place every time, as the woman whose house it is may tend to become the leader. Use as many different homes as possible. It is important to ensure that the meeting will not be interrupted or overheard, because as time goes on some women may wish to talk about very personal matters. It will also be necessary to

63

decide how long the meetings are going to last – about two hours is usual, once a week or once a fortnight.

It is important to agree on a structure for the meetings, as soon as possible. It is usually a good idea to have a leader for each meeting. Try to ensure that every member is encouraged to take a turn at this. Some women may find this task quite difficult, and it is important for the group to offer support to the woman who is leading that meeting. The task of this woman is to keep the group to the agreed programme, to start and finish the meeting on time, and to ensure that every woman has a chance to speak and be listened to. Whatever else happens in a meeting, time for chat will obviously be an important part because this will help the group to gel; so it is a good idea to keep at least half an hour at the beginning or end of each meeting for chat, leaving the rest of the time free to concentrate on whatever else is on the programme.

The programme for the meetings may be planned several meetings in advance, or decided at the end of each meeting. This all sounds very formal, but meetings will not be as enjoyable and useful as they could be unless there is an agreed structure, at least for a start until people get to know each other.

Another matter to be discussed at the beginning of a group is confidentiality. Some of the discussions which take place will be very personal, and everyone will feel more secure in a self-help group if it is possible to trust the members not to pass on personal information outside the group.

The length of a group's existence is another matter for decision. Will the group run for an agreed number of meetings and then finish, or will it continue? Some women prefer a limited time commitment, and the group's life can always be extended by agreement at the time if members wish to continue meeting. This avoids the problem of a group 'fading out'.

At one of the first meetings it is important that every member of the group should have an opportunity to talk about herself. This is likely to include where she is at in her menopause if it has started, and what her experiences have been so far. Some women are shy, so it is very important that others encourage them to talk. It is also necessary to give the woman who is talking full attention. During a discussion one golden rule is never to allow more than one conversation to take place at a time. The aim should be for every woman to have an equal chance to talk. This may mean that some women have to be asked to be quiet while someone else is talking. If you find that someone else's behaviour is upsetting or annoying you in the group, it is better to say so at the time, rather than to bottle it up. It is very important for women to have a mutual respect for each other and to be honest if the group is to be successful. In order to encourage this, some groups have a time for 'unfinished business' at the end of a meeting in order to clear up any misunderstandings or hurt feelings which may have occurred during the meeting, so that everyone looks forward to the next meeting.

When the group settles down, the members should decide whether or not it will remain open to new members. It is usually difficult for a group to develop a trusting atmosphere if members are always coming and going. One solution to this is to accept new members only from time to time.

WHAT TO TALK ABOUT?

The group will need to decide on topics or themes for discussion. In a menopause group this is usually not difficult because there is so much to talk about.

If the group is not sure what it wants to discuss, then ideas can be obtained through books. For example, some of the topics raised in this book could be discussed, taking a different one each time. It is better to avoid the temptation to invite outside experts in to speak to the group. You will find that, if the members are given encouragement, they will have a lot to offer each other, and the expertise will grow within the group.

Everyone's viewpoint is valid, even if other people do not agree or feel the same. It is helpful if the group can encourage its members to talk about how they *feel*. If someone gets upset, it is usually better to encourage her to have a good cry and let her feelings out, rather than immediately comforting her and trying to make her feel better. Sometimes it is better to express and live with uncomfortable and distressing feelings, with the support and care of other people, if we are to find a real solution for them.

Don't be discouraged if a group takes some time to get going. It takes time for people to get to know each other and have confidence to share feelings.

Some groups which become well established may be interested

in moving into a more wide-ranging kind of self-help therapy group. A very helpful book on this is *In Our Own Hands*, which suggests lots of exercises for self-help groups (see p.102).

Other self-help groups develop into pressure groups which try to improve local services for women, or perhaps encourage the setting-up of other menopause groups or women's health support groups. Whatever kind of group you are involved in, make sure you inform the Women's Health Information Centre (see p.102). In turn they will provide you with any local contacts they have listed.

CHECKLIST FOR SETTING UP A SELF-HELP GROUP
(1) Advertise group.
(2) Find 5–9 interested women.
(3) Arrange a meeting to discuss setting up a group.
(4) Find accommodation, decide length and times of group.
(5) Agree programme, and structure of meetings.

Points to remember
(1) Share leadership.
(2) Share speaking time as equally as possible between group members.
(3) Encourage everyone to join in.
(4) Listen to each other attentively.
(5) Keep confidentiality.

8 · HORMONE REPLACEMENT THERAPY

Hormone replacement therapy, or HRT, is based on the idea that, as the body's production of oestrogen and progesterone is reduced at the menopause, it should be possible to replace the lost hormones by substitutes or 'replacements', and thereby avoid the changes which might take place as the body adjusts to lowered levels of naturally-produced hormones.

We are neither promoting nor opposing the use of HRT, but feel that women should know the risks as well as the advantages so that they can make an informed choice. This is especially important as HRT is a form of treatment which is being increasingly promoted by some specialists. There is no doubt that HRT has a place in helping some women with particular problems. The purpose of this chapter is to look at the kinds of preparations which are available and consider the pros and cons for taking them.

NATURAL HORMONES

Hormone replacement therapy attempts to substitute for our naturally-produced oestrogen and progesterone. These hormones are responsible for our menstrual cycle, and also for the development of breasts, fertility, pregnancy and production of breast milk. Oestrogens also seem to play a part in the condition of the lining of the vagina, the lips and the vaginal opening or vulva, and tissues around the bladder. Two other hormones, follicle-stimulating hormone (FSH) and luteinising hormone (LH), produced by the pituitary gland in the brain, interact with the female hormones in a delicately balanced feedback system which regulates the amounts of oestrogen and progesterone produced. At the time of the approach of menopause the amounts of FSH and LH begin to increase and the levels of the sex hormones (oestrogen and progesterone) decrease. As progesterone and oestrogen are responsible for more than just the menstrual cycle, the menopause may be accompanied by other changes in addition to the ending of menstruation. Each woman is unique in the amounts of hormones she has produced during her cycles so that her body will have its own particular way of reacting when the sex hormones are reduced.

After the menopause, our bodies still produce oestrogens from body fat, the adrenal glands, and also from our ovaries – which is why it is important to keep them even if a hysterectomy has been necessary. Contrary to what some people say, oestrogen production does *not* stop after the menopause although the level of production is of course lower. There is still sufficient natural oestrogen circulating in the body for there to be very little change in body tissue, so vaginal dryness should not be a problem for the majority of women.

The actions on the body of natural progesterone and oestrogen are listed below:

Hormone	*Action*
Oestrogen	Development and maintenance of female sex organs, breasts. Maintenance of moistness of vagina.
Progesterone	Follows on from action of oestrogen on the lining of the uterus and brings about the period if there is no pregnancy. Prepares the uterus to receive the fertilised egg. Development of breasts. Maintenance of pregnancy.

THE MEDICAL USE OF HORMONES

In the early days of HRT the emphasis was on replacing oestrogen, and the first HRT preparations did not contain any progesterone-like substances. However it has been found that it is safer to include both to avoid cancer, and newer treatments include both. This is thought to be more like the natural situation of the menstrual cycle.

If you take oestrogen by itself, this is called 'unopposed' oestrogen and you will not have a monthly bleed. Taking a combination of oestrogen and progesterone means that the oestrogen is 'opposed'. In this case progesterone causes the lining of the uterus walls to break down and shed in a monthly bleed similar to menstruation. This prevents the build-up and thickening of the womb lining, and avoids the changes in cells and tissues which could possibly lead to cancer.

A woman doctor who has written fully about HRT has described it as 'blunderbuss treatment' because each woman's levels of hormones are unique. The amounts used in HRT preparations cannot ever be the same as the sensitive ups and downs of sex hormones circulating in each individual body. However, there are situations where substitution may be especially helpful, such as after the artificial menopause (see pp.78–9).

The generally accepted reasons given by doctors for prescribing HRT are the following:

(1) To relieve menopausal symptoms such as sweats, flushes and vaginal dryness.
(2) To slow down the process of thinning bones which increases after the menopause.
(3) To relieve the same symptoms which may occur after part or complete removal of the ovaries, or in some cases after hysterectomy when the ovaries may have stopped or suddenly reduced oestrogen production.

It should be noted that there is much argument within the medical profession about the rate of bone loss after menopause, and the effectiveness of HRT in slowing it down, and preventing osteoporosis.

It should also be noted that a doctor may not always make it clear why HRT is being prescribed, e.g. many women believe they have been given hormone treatment to help them sleep or 'cope' better. On the other hand, some women may not even be told that they are being given hormones at all.

Oestrogen *can* reduce sweats and hot flushes, and, if these are causing insomnia, tiredness and anxiety or other distress, they can generally improve the way a woman feels. HRT either by mouth in tablet form, or as a cream applied to the vagina, *can* help dry vaginal conditions.

HRT may be given to slow down the naturally-occurring bone loss which increases for a few years after the menopause, or to reduce other signs such as sweats, flushes or vaginal dryness which may occur after an early menopause, whether natural or as a result of surgery.

Although HRT may be prescribed to prevent bone loss and eventual osteoporosis, it is not clear how effective this really is and whether the risks outweigh the benefits. In any case scientific evidence shows that Vitamin D, diet, exercise and exposure to sunlight are all involved in bone health.

WHAT HRT CANNOT DO

Oestrogens prescribed around the menopause cannot prevent the natural process of ageing; although, because oestrogen can cause the body to store more fluid, it can puff the skin out which can stretch it and may thus appear to 'reduce' wrinkles. This is why it has earned a false reputation for being a rejuvenating or youth-preserving drug. The problem is that too much stored fluid in the tissues can lead to fluid retention and a bloated feeling. HRT cannot reverse osteoporosis and make the bones fully recover if the condition is already advanced. HRT is not effective in treating depression (but may help exhaustion and irritability if this has been brought on by loss of sleep resulting from severe night sweats). Men suffer from more coronary heart disease than women until about the age of 50 when both sexes are at the same risk – but it is not established that oestrogens given as HRT will protect women from heart disease. The use of oestrogen and progesterone replacement therapy will not increase sexual interest, though other sex hormone preparations containing androgens like testosterone (male hormone) have been tried in women for this purpose.

GUIDELINES FOR TAKING HRT

A lot more is known about the risks of HRT than when the first preparations came onto the market, and anyone considering using it should take into account the following guidelines:

(1) Take the smallest dosage which will relieve symptoms for the shortest possible time.
(2) Do not increase the dosage without medical advice.
(3) Take it under regular and careful supervision.
(4) Take a combination product and not oestrogen alone.
(5) After 6 or 12 months the dosage should be reduced and by the end of 2 years treatment should be discontinued.

(6) Never stop taking it suddenly but reduce dosage over a period of time under medical supervision, or your sweats, flushes and vaginal symptoms may return quite strongly.

(7) Take HRT only if you really feel you need it.

SEEING THE DOCTOR ABOUT HRT

If you do decide to take HRT you will need to have a thorough medical examination, which should include the following:

(1) An internal examination of the uterus and cervix – with a cervical smear if necessary.

(2) Blood pressure check.

(3) Breast examination.

(4) Urine tests.

The doctor should also take a note about your menstrual cycles and any experience you have had of breast cysts or lumpiness. There are a number of reasons for *not* taking HRT. These are:

(1) Known or suspected cancer of the uterus or breast.

(2) Abnormal bleeding which has not been investigated.

(3) Liver or gall bladder disease.

(4) Any past or present occurrence of thrombosis (blood clots).

A doctor should also ask about family health and whether there is a history of cancer of the breast or uterus. It may be inadvisable for you to take HRT if you have severe varicose veins, high blood pressure, kidney disease, diabetes, epilepsy and fibroids, or if you are overweight or a smoker. All these add to the risks of HRT. Because oestrogens can cause blood clotting they are not recommended if you have sickle cell trait or disease, but medical advice should be taken. You should also stop taking oestrogen several weeks before any major surgery because of its effect on blood clotting.

QUESTIONS TO ASK YOUR DOCTOR

(1) What medical checks on my health will you carry out?

(2) What checks will I need to do myself?

(3) Which kind of preparation will I be taking?

(4) Should I expect a period?

(5) Are there any particular side-effects you would like me to report to you?

(6) How long do you think I will be on the treatment?

(7) When should I return to see you?

TYPES OF TREATMENT

The preparations which are used for hormone replacement therapy are most frequently in tablet form. However, some oestrogens are also available as implants (pellets) which are put under the skin. There are also creams containing oestrogen and these are sometimes prescribed to help vaginal dryness.

Preparations in tablet form are available as oestrogen only, and in combined or 'sequential' form. Taking a sequential preparation means that during a 28-day cycle you will be receiving some oestrogen every day and some progestogen (progesterone substitute) during part of the cycle. As it is now known that the risk of cancer of the lining of the womb is decreased if a sequential preparation is taken, these products are listed first in Table 1.

Table 1: Sequential Preparations

Preparation	Oestrogen	Progestogen	Number of days of progestogen
Cycle-progynova	Oestradiol valerate	Levonorgestrel	10
Menophase	Mestranol	Norethisterone	13
Prempack	Conjugated Equine Oestrogens	Norgestrel	7
Prempack C	Conjugated Equine Oestrogens	Norgestrel	12
Trisequens	Oestradiol Oestriol	Norethisterone Acetate	10

If you are thinking of taking an HRT preparation, from the point of view of safety there are two major factors to consider. The addition of a progestogen to oestrogen does not by itself protect the body (especially the womb, but possibly also the breasts) from the risk of cancer. It is considered safest if progestogen is taken for not less than 10 days of each 28-day cycle.

The *type* of oestrogen in the preparation is also a factor when thinking about safety. The oestrogens which are described as 'natural' are known to carry less risk of thrombosis. Although Menophase includes a progestogen for 13 days of the cycle, its oestrogen Mestranol is not 'natural', and therefore it may cause greater changes in the way the blood clots, and carry a greater risk of thrombosis.

Table 2: Preparations Without Progestogens

Preparation	Oestrogen	Other hormones
Harmogen	Conjugated oestrogens ('natural' oestrogens)	
Hormonin	Oestrone, oestriol ('natural' oestrogens)	
Pentovis	Quinestradol (synthetic oestrogen)	
Mixogen	Ethinyl oestradiol (synthetic)	Methyl testosterone (androgen)
Estrovis	Quinestrol (synthetic)	

IMPLANTS

Implants are used sometimes after hysterectomy, partly to avoid some of the side-effects of taking oestrogen by mouth. However, if severe side-effects do occur, the implant has to be removed and this can be very difficult. If you have had an implant you *must* also take progestogen to protect the womb against the risk of cancer. Norethisterone (Primolut-N) or medroxyprogesterone (Provera) are sometimes used. This would then be similar to having combined therapy. Some women find that they frequently forget to take the tablets and this makes the implants less safe.

CREAMS

Oestrogen creams carry all the risks of, and can produce the same side-effects as, tablets with oestrogen. The oestrogen passes into the bloodstream from the vagina and long-term use is not recommended. Medical checks are just as necessary if you are using oestrogen in cream form as when you are using tablets or an implant.

SIDE-EFFECTS

If you have a womb, the sequential preparations will produce bleeding like a light period. This does not mean that you are having periods again, but that the uterus is reacting to the end of the progestogen treatment each month. Other side-effects include breast tenderness, weight gain, nausea, and PMT feelings. These should have subsided after two months, though if not it is usually a sign that the oestrogen dose is too high and another preparation could be tried. However, it is not usually considered worth trying more than two different preparations.

If you decide to take HRT, it is worth considering carefully, and discussing with your doctor, which preparation provides an effective dose and is the least risky.

If you start treatment it is important to:

(1) Check your breasts each month (after your 'period') if you are taking both oestrogen and a progestogen (which produces a monthly bleed). There are leaflets showing how to do this (see p.103).

(2) Note *any* side-effects. Write them down and tell your doctor.

(3) Have your blood pressure checked at least once a month after the first few months of treatment.

(4) Take note of any irregular bleeding and go back to your doctor should it occur.

(5) Understand the type of treatment you are being given – that is whether it is oestrogen alone, or includes a progestogen. If you are taking oestrogen alone and haven't had a hysterectomy then the risk of cancer of the uterus lining (endometrium) is greater and you will need a D and C (scrape) at least every two years. Even if you have had a hysterectomy, you will still need to check your breasts regularly each month.

OTHER HORMONE PREPARATIONS

Progestogens alone, for example medroxyprogesterone and nor-ethisterone, have been used to relieve hot flushes and night sweats. However progestogens have side-effects which include depression,

74

acne, breast tenderness and weight gain. Sometimes a hormone preparation might be prescribed which contains an androgen like methyltestosterone, and this is thought to increase sexual interest and libido.

OTHER PREPARATIONS

It would be useful to have a treatment which could reduce hot flushes and night sweats, if needed, without the use of hormones which have a certain amount of risk. One such preparation, clonidine, has been tried. It is generally used for treating high blood pressure and has side-effects which include drowsiness.

There are other measures which can reduce the effects of the menopause without the risk attached to HRT, such as improving diet, taking exercise and looking after yourself (see Chapter 9).

9 · HEALTH IN MID-LIFE – SOME SELF-HELP SUGGESTIONS

This chapter is a self-help guide to understanding and dealing with various problems which affect our health. Many of them are often mistakenly linked to the menopause, as if it were an illness. Some of the effects listed below *are* directly related to the menopause, e.g. night sweats, and these in turn may lead to such problems as fatigue due to loss of sleep.

Other health problems which occur in mid-life, and at other times, are due to the stresses and domestic changes we talked about in Chapters 3 and 4. Others again, e.g. joint and muscle pains, can be effects of ageing. Life-style, diet, exercise, alcohol and smoking also affect our general wellbeing – throughout our lives.

The topics listed below are in alphabetical order so that you can dip into the chapter and read the parts which interest you.

ABSENT-MINDEDNESS
See Poor Concentration; Exhaustion.

ANXIETY
(See also Depression; Stress.) Women and men can experience anxiety or panic attacks – those sudden feelings of dread which seem to come out of the blue! They may follow, or be accompanied by sweating, flushing, or palpitations (a sudden increase in the rate of heartbeat, or fluttery sensations in the chest). These sensations are not dangerous but you should check with your doctor if you experience chest pains, especially if you smoke. The anxiety feelings and palpitations pass in a few minutes. Occasionally some people may continue to feel a bit low in spirits, or the vague anxiety hangs around for a little longer.

These anxiety or panic feelings may have a number of possible causes: body temperature changes which also accompany hot flushes and sweats; smoking cigarettes; things we eat and drink, e.g. coffee, strong tea, sugar, alcohol, salt, food additives (such as monosodium glutamate [MSG]: it's in many foods – check the labels!); lack of exercise (sluggish circulation or digestion, etc); stress or worries which we haven't recognised or dealt with; withdrawal from some drugs such as tranquillisers can also produce anxiety or panic feelings.

REMEDIES

(1) Try to cut out or cut down on salt intake, cigarettes, tea, coffee, alcohol, sugar, unnecessary food additives like monosodium glutamate (sometimes called 'flavour enhancer' on food packets).

(2) Check with your doctor if you are taking any medicines. Your panic or anxiety might be a side-effect. Avoid taking tranquillisers if you possibly can.

(3) Check your diet. Make sure you are getting sufficient calcium, which has a natural calming and relaxing effect, and can aid sleep if taken at night before you go to bed as a hot milk drink. Also make sure you are getting sufficient Vitamin B Complex which is particularly important for preventing stress and promoting a healthy digestive and nervous system. Vitamin preparations should be taken at the recommended dosage. Vitamin B6, in particular, is dangerous in too high doses. (See Vitamins.)

(4) Make sure you are looking after *yourself* as well as those around you. For example:

(a) Make some time each day to relax and develop the habit of allowing yourself some regular peace and quiet just to do whatever pleases *you*.

(b) Do some deep breathing/relaxation exercises.

(c) Think about joining a class or group to try something new that you would enjoy or find interesting – either on your own, or with a partner or friend.

(d) Share your feelings with your women friends – they might welcome the chance to talk to you in turn and you can support each other if you feel low, or worried.

(e) Learn to give and receive relaxing massage with your partner or a friend.

77

(f) Contact a counsellor or therapist if you feel you would like to talk to someone else about things you feel might be causing the stress or anxiety.

BLADDER PROBLEMS

See Bloatedness; Constipation; Stress Incontinence; Vaginal Changes.

BLEEDING

(See also Irregular Periods.) A common indication of the approach of menopause is irregular bleeding. Periods can become lighter or heavier; and more or less frequent, with erratic gaps between them. Irregular bleeding can also be caused by polyps, or fibroids, or oestrogen in oral contraceptives or hormone replacement therapy. If heavy bleeding is experienced before the menopause, it should always be investigated by your doctor, and so should *any* bleeding after the menopause (unless you are receiving HRT in a combined form – oestrogen *with* a progestogen – which is designed to include a monthly bleed). It is probably nothing serious but it could be an indication of infection, fibroids or cancer. Early treatment is important to deal with these effectively.

REMEDIES

Medical treatments for heavy bleeding or flooding include treatment with hormones (which can have side-effects such as bloatedness, nausea, headaches and weight gain); a D and C (when the lining of the womb is scraped under a general anaesthetic); or a hysterectomy (when the womb or part of it is removed in a major operation).

If your doctor suggests a hysterectomy, you may like to get in touch with someone from The Hysterectomy Self Help and Support Group (see p.104), who will discuss it with you to help you decide whether you wish to take this major step. If you do decide you need to have your womb removed you should make sure that your ovaries are *not* also removed unless they themselves are actually diseased in some way, and it is therefore absolutely necessary. They are important organs before, during and after the menopause as they continue to produce hormones (oestrogen and androgens) needed by your body. If it is necessary for your ovaries to be removed, you may experience an immediate and quite severe menopause if you haven't already gone through it naturally. And it may be necessary for you to have a course of hormone replacement therapy (HRT) while your body adapts itself to an altered hormone pattern.

OTHER TREATMENTS FOR HEAVY FLOW
Vitamin C Complex (found in the peel and white pulp of citrus fruits – so eat some of the white pith and pulp of your daily orange or grapefruit, and green peppers).

N.B. If you have been losing large amounts of blood, you may also have some anaemia. This needs supervised treatment so consult your doctor for a proper check-up and appropriate treatment. Over-the-counter remedies can be expensive, ineffective, and produce other problems such as constipation and gastric upsets.

BLOATEDNESS
(See also Constipation; Stress Incontinence.) Some women may suffer from puffiness, swelling or bloated feelings. These might be in the face, breasts, hands, stomach or pelvic regions, legs, ankles or feet, and may be accompanied by a headache, especially in the morning. It may be because extra fluid is collecting in body tissues: this is known as 'fluid retention' and, if extreme, needs supervised medical treatment. Medical evidence suggests that jobs involving long periods of sitting or standing still may contribute to or even cause fluid retention. It can also result from taking hormones in oral contraceptives or hormone replacement therapy, certain anti-depressants, or analgesics; and from too much salt in your diet. It can also be related to hormone fluctuation during the menstrual cycle; and be affected by hot weather temperatures.

REMEDIES
(1) If you are on hormones discuss the suitability of your treatment with your doctor.
(2) Cut down on the salt in your diet.
(3) Eat foods which are natural diuretics (increase your urine output) e.g. cabbage, cucumber, celery (especially in juice form), parsley, watermelon, grapes, fresh pineapple, asparagus, parsnips, watercress, melon, strawberries, cranberries.

(4) If you are using these natural diuretics and your urine output *is* increased, you also need to eat foods which are rich in potassium, e.g. bananas, oranges, soya beans, peaches, apricots, dates, figs, prunes, raisins.

(5) Vitamin B6 (pyridoxine) is often prescribed to women who suffer from pre-menstrual tension (PMT) to relieve bloat symptoms. Try it for a month or so at a dose of 30–50 mg per day. If this doesn't seem to make any difference, try another month at 50–80 mg per day. It is possible to take higher doses, but it would be best to discuss it with your doctor as higher doses, for longer periods, can be dangerous and cause serious side-effects. Vitamin B6 occurs in yeast, liver, cereals, meat and other foods.

N.B. Women with Parkinson's Disease who are receiving L-Dopa should not take Vitamin B6 because it reduces the action of L-Dopa.

(6) Oil of Evening Primrose is prescribed by some specialists for PMT. It can also be bought in health food shops but is very expensive.

Fluid retention is frequently associated with a complaint known as 'irritable' bowel or colon, which is characterised by flatulence (wind), abdominal pain, and constipation alternating with diarrhoea. An appropriate diet will help you to keep the condition under control – see the dietician at your local hospital or health centre.

BONE PROBLEMS

(See also Osteoporosis; Joint Pains.) There is considerable discussion within the medical profession as to what causes osteoporosis (brittle bones). Although no-one can say for sure why some women develop osteoporosis in later life and others don't, it is clear that this condition which occurs after calcium is lost over a long period of time from the bones, is influenced by diet, smoking, exercise and exposure of the skin to sunlight (which produces Vitamin D), and oestrogens. Bone loss speeds up after menopause. Whether this becomes a serious problem or not could depend on the state of our bones at the time of the menopause, and what steps we then take to counteract calcium loss.

PREVENTIVE MEASURES

(1) Give up smoking! Women who smoke may be more prone to osteoporosis.

(2) Don't diet severely or continuously. Don't eat a continual very high protein diet: vegetarians appear to experience less osteoporosis.

(3) To counteract calcium loss women over 35 years of age should be taking in about 1 g of calcium per day. From 45, or when the menopause occurs if this is earlier, the amount should be increased to 1.5 g per day. The body requires a sufficient amount of Vitamin D to help it absorb calcium properly. Vitamin D can be stored in the body: a good amount of exposure to the sun during the summer will probably last you until late autumn. During winter and spring eat Vitamin D rich foods regularly once a week, such as herring, kippers, mackerel, sardines, eggs, as well as fortified cereals and margarines. Most people should not need extra Vitamin D. However, if you can't tolerate oily fish or sunlight, or are housebound, the recommended daily dose is between 2.5 and 10 micrograms (100–400 international units). Halibut liver oil capsules contain Vitamin D. Too much Vitamin D can be dangerous. Calcium-rich foods are spinach, spring greens, kale, watercress, endive, yoghourt, buttermilk, cheese, and sesame seeds (or tahini, which is a 'butter' made out of crushed sesame seeds) – half a cup of them = 580 mg calcium. Gently roasting them helps you digest them. Put them in the bottom of a saucepan over a lowish heat until they go a golden brown, shaking them so that they don't burn. Let them go cold, and put them in a screwtop jar. Sprinkle them over your morning cereal, or over salads. Use them in cakes or biscuits, or with honey on bread. Milk is also a very good source of calcium: 1 pint of skimmed milk provides 761 mg; semi-skimmed milk = 729 mg; full cream milk = 702 mg; (See Appendix 4 for table of high-calcium foods.)

(4) Exercise: it is known that calcium leaks very quickly from unused bones. Exercise can prevent bones from softening, and can help to strengthen them. Exercise should be against gravity – brisk walking (say 30 minutes per day three days a week and more if you can fit it in), dancing, jogging, skipping, and any games or most sports. Swimming on its own is not sufficient. Although very good for keeping the body flexible and exercised it doesn't exercise the bones.

BREATHLESSNESS

The most obvious causes of breathlessness are cigarette smoking, or being overweight. The feeling of needing air may precede or accompany a hot flush, or be a reaction to tension or stress. Or it may be a sign of insufficient exercise – especially of the lungs and chest.

REMEDIES

(1) Stop smoking or try to cut down considerably.
(2) Lose some weight.
(3) Wear loose, light clothes so that you can take them off and put them back on again more easily if you are having sweats or flushes.
(4) Try to do some regular relaxation exercises during the day.
(5) Make sure you do something each day that makes you 'puff' – like running for a bus, walking upstairs, walking very briskly up slopes so that your lungs and chest area are expanded and exercised at least once a day. Better still, try to take up a regular activity which will improve your breathing, such as swimming or yoga.

N.B. If you experience pains in the chest as well as breathlessness, check with your doctor. It is a good idea to do this anyway before you start any strenuous activity if you haven't been active for a while.

CHILLS

Some women often feel cold and shivery after a hot flush or sweat. This passes in a few minutes, but it helps if you wear 'layers' of clothing so that you can peel off quickly when the flush or sweat begins, and then replace them as it begins to fade to avoid the extremes of body temperature changes.

CONSTIPATION

(See also Bloatedness; Stress Incontinence.) Constipation can produce cramps, distended bloated feelings and painful tenderness in the pelvic region. This can either be because of the actual hard mass in the bowel, or because of trapped wind.

Constipation can be caused by diet, dehydration, lack of exercise, stress, hormonal changes (some women are constipated regularly each month before their menstruation), or be a side-effect of medicines which contain codeine, decongestants which dry out cold symptoms, and some tranquillisers.

If you are experiencing vaginal or urinary tenderness during your menopause, it may be that the general inflammation or tenderness in the pelvic area is also causing constipation.

Constipation should not be ignored or just accepted: it can lead to more serious and troublesome complaints, such as irritable bowel or colon, and colitis.

REMEDIES

(1) Make sure you get enough fibre in your diet (whole wheat cereals, bread and flour, etc) as well as plenty of fresh fruit and raw vegetables. Don't eat uncooked bran; it can increase your calcium loss!

(2) Drink more water, *especially* if you increase your fibre intake as it soaks up more moisture while you are digesting it, and can then make constipation worse!

(3) Nourish the lining of the bowel by taking yoghourt (live, not processed), buttermilk, acidophilus – all of which helps the bowel to do its work more effectively.

(4) Take more exercise – like walking. Swimming is especially good for exercising the internal parts of the body as well as muscles. Learn yoga or some abdomen-stretching exercises.

(5) Try to pinpoint and deal with any stressful factors in your life, although this may be easier said than done!

(6) Don't take decongestants or painkillers (headache tablets, etc) unless you *really* need them – or ask your doctor to help you work out a better regime if you need drugs or medication on a regular basis. Ask if constipation is a side-effect of what you are given.

(7) Don't use liquid paraffin or commercial laxatives unless specifically prescribed by your doctor. Natural laxatives are an alternative; try black molasses, prunes (stewed or juice), cider-vinegar, honey, raw fruit and vegetables, salads or muesli.

(8) Lie on your back with your legs stretched out and massage your stomach gently in the morning before you get out of bed.

(9) When you want to pass a motion, sit on the lavatory with your feet on something to raise your knees in front of you so that you don't strain yourself.

DEPRESSION

(See also Anxiety; Stress.) Most women suffer from depression at some time or another. Sometimes we feel a bit low for a few hours. At other times it may last for days, weeks, or even sometimes years, and be like a cloud on top of us, which affects the whole of our life.

Recent studies show that depression is brought on by ordinary events in women's lives, for example having several young children to care for; or not having anyone to confide in. Many of us feel guilty when we think we are not coping with ordinary everyday life, so the feelings of dissatisfaction, resentment, anger and power-lessness, which are natural responses to stressful situations, get pushed down and bottled up instead of being acknowledged and dealt with. This may make us feel hopeless, despairing, weepy, exhausted; in other words, depressed.

Although there is no evidence that women are more liable to be depressed around the time of the menopause, it is as well to be aware of three things. The first is that changes in hormone levels can cause mood changes (as is well known by women who suffer from PMT). These may occur for some women as a result of fluctuating hormones, especially in the two to three years immediately before the menopause.

Secondly, there are plenty of stresses and changes taking place in mid-life which might lead us to feel depressed. They may also have the opposite effect of making us feel angry. Anger is a good cure for depression, although most of us do not find it easy to express our feelings in this way – we have been taught for too long to believe that it is 'unladylike'.

Thirdly, many people mistakenly assume that menopause causes us to become mentally unstable. It is easy to fall in with other people's assumptions, and expect to feel under the weather. We may then find ourselves using the menopause as an excuse for feeling depressed. If we do this, it will prevent us from discovering and dealing with the real causes of our depression.

One of the features of depression is that it makes us feel worthless, guilty and hopeless. This often makes us reluctant to seek help. We are more likely to stay in bed or shut ourselves in the house. The most important thing to do when we are feeling depressed is to share our feelings with others – to talk. Unfortunately doctors do not usually have much time to talk to their patients, so they often prescribe drugs for people who are depressed.

A short course of anti-depressant drug treatment sometimes enables people to get over the worst feelings of depression or anxiety, and to start working at whatever is causing the depression. But it is very important to be wary of becoming dependent on tranquillisers: unfortunately, some doctors prescribe them very freely, and may even write repeat prescriptions without seeing their patients. Although tranquillisers were previously thought not to be addictive, it is now recognised that many are. Tranquillisers are certainly not a long-term solution to people's problems.

There are organisations which help people who are addicted, and some are listed on pp.107–8.

REMEDIES

(1) The best way of dealing with depression is to talk to other people. Sometimes, it will be enough to phone or meet a friend or go out with other people. If the depression is more than a passing mood, it is important to find someone you can talk to about how awful you are feeling. Talking and sharing may begin to identify what is making you feel depressed and make it possible to start looking for a way of bringing about changes in your life. There is sometimes a point where friends may not be able to help any further. Indeed you may even risk losing friends by demanding too much of them. At this stage it may be necessary to find a sympathetic and understanding person who is trained to help you sort out the possible causes of your depression. There is a list of sources of help on p.108, but a good standby is the local branch of the Samaritans, or your local 'Mind'. Some areas have walk-in crisis centres.

(2) Don't blame yourself. There is a good reason for your depression which is not your fault.

(3) Allow yourself to be angry. Other people may not like you being angry, but it will release some energy which will help you to take action, and that will make you feel better.

(4) Take care of yourself.

(5) Join a women's discussion or health group.

(6) Try a 'Stress Relaxation' type of course at your local Adult Institute.

(7) Read one of the very helpful books on depression (see p.108).

DIZZINESS

If you experience dizzy feelings, you should have a check-up with your doctor to make sure your blood pressure is normal. Dizziness may be nothing to do with the menopause, but could be related to a number of other factors: the side-effects of medicines (like tranquillisers or sleeping pills), or the result of dieting. When you experience dizziness, just sit quietly for a few minutes, relax and breathe regularly, and it will pass.

DYSPAREUNIA (Painful Intercourse)

See Vaginal Changes; Libido.

EXHAUSTION

(See also Stress.) Many women feel tired and exhausted. This is hardly surprising given the number of jobs and tasks that most women have to do day in and day out, both inside and outside the home! Overweight or an underactive thyroid can both result in feelings of exhaustion. Sleepless nights caused by sweats and flushes can also lead to feelings of exhaustion.

REMEDIES

(1) Make sure everyone else you live with is doing their share of the chores and household tasks. Men can 'retire' from their jobs or 'rest' at the end of the day's work: women are expected to go on for ever! Don't wait on children – make sure they know how to look after themselves and take their fair share of domestic responsibility.

(2) Try to relax in your lunch hour if you also work outside the home. Many women expect or are expected to shop or do the washing in their lunch hour. Delegate as much as possible to others. Don't let people at work take advantage of you.

(3) Some women have isolated waves of exhaustion during or immediately after a flush or sweat – just sit and relax, it will pass.

(4) Join an assertiveness training course: they are enjoyable, interesting, and help you to get your needs met without having rows or arguments.

(5) Very occasionally an underactive thyroid gland can be the cause of tiredness. This should be checked with your doctor.

FATIGUE

See Exhaustion.

FLATULENCE

(See also Constipation; Bloatedness.) Wind or gas in the bowels can often be a deeply worrying and embarrassing problem, as well as being extremely painful. It can interfere with a woman's social, working and emotional life. Stress can underly it, through causing bad digestion. Or it may be an allergy to certain common foods eaten daily. Or a 'lazy' colon or 'irritable' bowel could have developed through prolonged constipation or diarrhoea, due to indigestion, bad diet, stress, lack of exercise because of sedentary job etc, or the side-effects of drugs.

REMEDIES

(1) Read a good health book which has a chapter on constipation, irritable bowel, flatulence, etc.
(2) Talk to your GP if s/he is sympathetic and will take you seriously.
(3) Make an appointment to see the dietician at your local health centre or hospital (you may need to get your doctor to refer you, but you could try phoning them direct yourself).
(4) Make sure you have fibre in your diet – use a high-fibre cereal, or muesli, or wholemeal bread or toast for breakfast each day. Also drink more fluid. Eat fresh fruit every day and lightly cooked vegetables (but go easy on cabbage and pulses for a while: although very good for you they can cause wind until your body gets used to them).
(5) Eat lots of live yoghourt – it's good for your bowel and digestive system.
(6) Try to reduce the stress factors in your life.
(7) Relax more – try to arrange your life to give space for you to please yourself in some way.

FLOODING

(See also Bleeding.) Heavy periods can be a sign of approaching menopause. They can also indicate a number of other problems and should always be investigated by your doctor.

FLUSHES AND SWEATS

Sometimes before, but usually after, the menopause, most women experience some degree of hot or cold sweats, and hot flushes. These can happen separately or together, and the patterns can vary. They are not dangerous at all. The flushes may range from a very slight blushing or warm sensation to huge waves of heat surging all over the upper part of the body and sometimes lower back, stomach and pelvic area, followed immediately by a faint mist of sweat around the upper lip and forehead, or a more drenching sweat breaking out all over the face and upper part of the body, soaking clothes or bedding. Frequently the flushing may not be visible so there is no need to worry or feel embarrassed about other people's reactions. Flushes can last from a few seconds to a few minutes, and can occur once or several times during a day or night. They often occur in phases, and may also be related to stress or worry or certain activities such as drinking strong coffee or smoking cigarettes.

Sometimes they may be accompanied by palpitations, slight nausea, or feelings of utter exhaustion for about three to five minutes or less. And sometimes they can be followed by chilled, shivery feelings for a few minutes.

Sweats can cause problems by disturbing sleep, especially if a partner is sharing the same bed.

REMEDIES

(1) Try not to worry or feel embarrassed. This may make them worse. Some women take the plunge and tell friends and family and even people they work with that they are menopausal, and need to be left alone for a minute or two if they have a hot flush or sweat, until it has passed. If this seems too difficult to deal with, try to relax and calm yourself: breathe deeply and regularly, and sit or lie quite still, as relaxed as possible.

(2) Dress in 'layers' so you can remove and replace something quickly and easily. Push sleeves up and rest inside of arms and wrists on something cold – go and put them under the cold tap. Stand in a cool air flow in a doorway or in front of a window.

(3) At night, leave the covers untucked if you haven't got a duvet. Fold them back from your body if you feel a sweat or flush coming on or are woken by one.

(4) Use cotton sheets, nightwear, and pillowcases if possible; avoid artificial fibres in your daytime clothing too, if possible. Cotton absorbs moisture more easily and makes it less likely that you will need to change the sheets in the night.

(5) If a partner is acting unsympathetically or uncooperatively, try sleeping by yourself occasionally to give you both a better night's sleep.

(6) Vitamin E therapy is very helpful for many women in reducing or stopping sweats and flushing. Take 200 iu (international units) Vitamin E per day for one month. If there is no improvement, increase the dose to 300 or 400 iu. Again, have patience and take it for three to four weeks. If this seems to do the trick, maintain the dose for two to three months and cut down to a lower level again. If this still works, decrease again. The idea is to try to get the lowest level which will prevent them occurring. If they come back, or don't seem to improve, you can increase the level. Your body needs three to four weeks to get used to each level of dosage, so have patience. Don't go above 600 iu per day in any case. Don't stay on Vitamin E indefinitely: have a month's break every now and then. Vitamin E is present in the oil from soya beans, wheat germ, rice germ, cotton seed, and maize, and is in green leaves. It does not appear to be destroyed by cooking.

N.B. Don't take Vitamin E if you have diabetes, rheumatic heart or high blood pressure, except in consultation with your doctor.

(7) Ginseng has also helped some women to cope with flushing and sweating, and it is supposed to be very helpful with vaginal dryness. (See under Vaginal Symptoms for more information.)

(8) Cut out or cut down on food and drinks that are stimulants: coffee, strong tea, spices, alcohol, etc, especially at night, and sugar.

(9) Try a warm milk drink last thing at night or a soothing herbal tea (camomile or one of the ones marketed for good sleep).

(10) Cut out or down on cigarettes – some women say they often have a hot flush just after the first puff of each cigarette!

(11) Talk to women friends. Join a menopause group or women's health group or class and share your feelings and experiences in a supportive, enjoyable atmosphere. Women in groups often feel very much better about their symptoms and life in general after a

good supportive discussion – and often a good laugh with other women going through the menopause.

(12) HRT may be necessary for a short time if you are experiencing very disturbed sleep and this is creating problems for you.

FORGETFULNESS

See Poor Concentration.

FORMICATION

This is the strange itchy sensation like ants crawling on the skin or inside the limbs. It can feel like pins and needles too. It is rather disagreeable and appears to be related to the circulation system, which may explain why some women experience it during the menopause.

REMEDIES

Make sure you get enough exercise. When it happens, try shaking or kicking your legs for a few minutes.

HEADACHES

(See also Migraine.) Some women have more headaches around the time of the menopause. These may be related to hormonal changes (causing fluid retention and bloatedness, for example). Or it may be the result of stress, or diet (food allergy), or a reaction to drugs.

REMEDIES

If they are very severe, or of long duration, they may be migraines. But it would be as well to check with your doctor in any case.

(1) Try to alleviate the stressful factors.

(2) Find a good book from your library or health food shop on food allergies and headaches.

(3) Consider visiting a homeopath, naturopath, or herbalist.

N.B. Some people develop osteoarthritis in middle age (not to be confused with osteoporosis or rheumatoid arthritis!). This could mean that they have a pinched or trapped nerve or tissue in their neck or spine which could be producing the headaches, as well as other unexplained sharp or shooting pains elsewhere in the body.

Posture is *crucial* in this case and learning to sit, lie and stand properly can often completely alleviate such pains. Osteopathy and Alexander Technique can be very helpful.

HEAVY PERIODS
See Bleeding.

HYSTERECTOMY
See pages 15 and 78–9.

INSOMNIA
(See Flushes and Sweats; Anxiety; Depression.) Insomnia may be caused by night sweats, resulting in disturbed sleep patterns, or worry about disturbing a partner if you are sharing a bed; or it may be related to anxiety or depression; or it may be caused by diet. Lack of exercise might contribute as well.

REMEDIES
Try to relax and not get too upset about it – this will make it worse.

(1) Cut out coffee and strong tea, cigarettes, sugar and alcohol, especially at night – although the occasional nightcap if you don't drink much can help.
(2) Learn some relaxation exercises and do them before you go to bed in the evening.
(3) Make sure you have some proper exercise each day – a brisk walk for 10–15 minutes will help (unless you are very active as a matter of course each day).
(4) Have a hot shower or bath before you go to bed.
(5) Relax with a good book for a while when you first get into bed.
(6) Take a hot milk drink or herbal night tea to bed.
(7) Learn to give and receive gentle relaxing massage with a partner or friend: stroke and soothe each other into calmness and relaxation.

If you feel desperate for sleep, you could try tranquillisers or sleeping tablets from your doctor, but only take them for a short time until you have got a sleeping pattern back – otherwise they can make matters far worse.

IRREGULAR PERIODS
(See also Bleeding.) This is a common sign of approaching meno-

pause, and apart from the inconvenience of being caught out unawares is nothing to worry about.

N.B. You should continue with contraception if you are in a heterosexual relationship and do not wish to become pregnant, until you have had no periods for at least a year. It is best not to use the pill as this interferes with your natural hormone production and disguises your real cycle, so you won't know when you are menopausal.

IRRITABILITY

(See also Anxiety; Depression; Exhaustion.) Some women feel irritable on occasions during the time around the menopause: fluctuating hormones can cause mood change as is well known with PMT. In addition, flushing and sweating, perhaps causing sleepless nights, can be very stressful. Some flushes produce feelings of complete exhaustion, making it difficult to cope if they coincide with someone making demands, however small. Women who would normally describe themselves as even-tempered or passive may experience sudden surges of irritation or even real rage at such a moment.

REMEDIES

Try to sort out whether the demands being made on you are *in any case* unreasonable, and try to get some help. For many women with heavy or taxing 'caring' duties, the fluctuating hormonal mood changes can feel like the last straw which finally makes coping impossible. Otherwise, if the feelings are fairly isolated, or less severe, try to relax more and look after yourself.

(1) Make sure you are getting enough calcium (it has a natural calming effect) and Vitamin B complex, which is good for the nervous system and general wellbeing.

(2) Cut out stimulating food and drink (cigarettes, strong tea, coffee, sugar, alcohol), and try to see if it is connected with any particular food you eat.

(3) Make sure it's not a side-effect of any drugs or medication you are taking: check with your doctor if you are on a regular medication.

ITCHY VULVA

(See also Vaginal Changes.) If you don't think it is connected with the menopause, check out the possibility that it is thrush, or NSU (non-specific urethritis), which is an infection of the vagina. The Health Education Council produces leaflets on these. The book *Our Bodies Ourselves* lists and gives ideas of how to deal with vaginal infections. If it is a severe problem for you, check with your doctor.

JOINT PAINS

(See also Bone Problems; Osteoporosis.) These may be related to menopausal activity and altering hormone levels, or to the natural ageing process, perhaps indicating the onset of some form of arthritis, or they may be caused by being overweight.

REMEDIES

(1) Make sure you sit and stand properly. Don't sit or stand for long periods of time without moving around or changing position.
(2) Try not to carry heavy loads especially in ways that pull your back unevenly.
(3) Make sure your bed doesn't sag: put a board under the mattress to make sure your body is in the correct position when you sleep, or buy an orthopaedic mattress if you can afford it. Don't have too thick a pillow. Don't slump in a chair when you relax – watching television or reading, etc; keep your back supported.
(4) Exercise is a crucial factor in preventing osteoporosis: not only does it prevent calcium leaking from the bones, but it also keeps the muscles and sinews around the bones and organs in better shape. Swimming and walking (without carrying heavy bags!) are two of the finest forms of exercise.
(5) Lose some weight if you are too heavy.
(6) Read a good book on the subject.
(7) If the pains are very severe or troublesome, check with your doctor.

LASSITUDE/LACK OF ENERGY

See Exhaustion; Flushes and Sweats.

LIBIDO

(See also Vaginal Changes.) Libido or sexual feelings can wax or wane for a number of reasons: no sexual partner; boredom or lack of interest in partner; partner's lack of interest; unsympathetic partner; tiredness; stress, anxiety or depression; hormonal fluctuations; side-effect of drugs; etc.

Sexual feelings can also revive after the menopause for women in heterosexual relationships because the fear of pregnancy is at last gone.

There are some good books now available on sexuality and you might be interested in finding out more on the subject, although many of them assume that either all women are married, or have a male partner. This can feel exclusive to celibate or lesbian women, or women living alone. Two books that cover most aspects of sexuality are *The Mirror Within Us* and *Women's Experience of Sex*. (See p.113 for full details.)

Masturbation for any woman, regardless of her circumstances, can be a relaxing and most enjoyable experience, although unfortunately many women have been raised to think that touching their own bodies is shameful or dirty in some way. Getting to know our own bodies can be a relaxing, releasing and positive experience and can help if a woman wants to increase her libido or sexual response feelings. It can also help women know what they would like their partner to do for them during love-making if they are in a relationship. If we learn to love ourselves a bit more, it can help with our self-esteem and self-confidence too.

If you are very worried about your sex life, get in touch with an experienced counsellor who specialises in sexual matters and sexual relationships of any kind. Try the Marriage Guidance Council – don't be put off by the name if you aren't married – they now have experienced counsellors on their staff who can help with any sort of sexual relationship or problem, or put you in touch with someone.

MIGRAINE

(See also Headaches.) If you think or know you are suffering from migraine, get in touch with The British Migraine Association, The Migraine Clinic, or The Migraine Trust. Migraine can be an allergic reaction to some foods. Or it can be a stress-related reaction. There are also some helpful books. (See Appendix 1.)

MOODINESS
See Anxiety; Depression; Irritability.

MUSCLE PAINS
See Joint Pains.

NAUSEA
Some women have occasional feelings of nausea, often at the same time as a hot flush. This is probably due to fluctuating hormones, rather like morning sickness in early pregnancy. It is nothing to worry about and usually passes very quickly.

NERVOUSNESS
See Anxiety; Depression; Irritability.

OSTEOPOROSIS
(See also Bone Problems; Joint Pains.) Osteoporosis is often linked to the menopause by some gynaecologists and specialists. They refer to the menopause as a 'deficiency disease' and suggest that all women should take hormone replacement therapy as a preventive measure, after the menopause. Although all women who live long enough will go through the menopause, only 20–25 per cent of them will ultimately develop severe osteoporosis and fractures. Nevertheless, this *is* a large minority, and all women should do what they can to protect themselves against it.

From continuing medical debate and research around the world, several factors are emerging. These are that diet (i.e. calcium and Vitamin D), exposure to sunlight (i.e. Vitamin D) and exercise are all crucially related in some way to hormonal activity and the building-up or breaking-down of bone. If there is insufficient calcium in the bloodstream, it is taken from bone to make up the loss. Calcium is lost from the body every day in the urine or excreta, and needs replacing daily.

PAINFUL INTERCOURSE
See Vaginal Changes.

PALPITATIONS
See Anxiety.

PANIC ATTACKS

See Anxiety.

POOR CONCENTRATION/ABSENT-MINDEDNESS/FORGETFULNESS

See also Exhaustion; Depression; Insomnia. As we saw in the section on ageing in Chapter 2, both men and women can begin to experience varying degrees of short-term memory loss as part of the human ageing process, and this can affect the efficiency of the long-term memory as well. Alternatively, it may be that you are overstressed or exhausted, and it's your body's way of saying 'enough'. Worrying about it could also make it worse.

PROLAPSE

See Stress Incontinence.

SCANTY PERIODS

See Bleeding; Irregular Periods.

SEXUAL RESPONSE

See Libido; Vaginal changes.

SEXUALITY

See Libido; Vaginal changes.

SLEEPLESSNESS

See Insomnia.

SORE VAGINA

See Vaginal Changes.

STRESS

(See also Anxiety; Depression.) Stress is a 'hidden' factor in most people's lives because it is often unrecognised or unacknowledged. The symptoms of stress, which can occur in people of any age and either sex, are very similar to those which are often said to be caused by the menopause. They include sweating, flushing, palpitations, exhaustion, breathlessness, headache, lack of sexual desire and insomnia amongst other things. People who are under stress behave in erratic ways, often being moody, weepy or irritable, and feeling anxious, depressed and unable to cope.

A certain amount of stress can be positive: it can keep us feeling alive, alert and on our toes. Too much is harmful and can damage our health and ability to function.

Ideally we need to be able to identify and eliminate the stressful things in our lives. Where this is not possible, we must learn to take care of ourselves to counteract and reduce the effects of stress.

STRESS INCONTINENCE

(See also Bladder Problems; Vaginal Changes.) Sometimes during middle age, and often before, women find that they begin to 'leak' urine if they cough, sneeze or laugh, etc. This is known as stress incontinence. It is caused by the deteriorating condition of the muscles and tissues in the pelvic cavity: lack of exercise, or exercise of the wrong sort, or perhaps childbirth has allowed them to become stretched or to lose their elasticity. Or it may be related to the menopause as well: perhaps the vaginal lining has become dry and sore – this can affect the bladder and the urethra (the tube we pass urine through), making us feel as though we've got cystitis and need to keep passing urine. If our pelvic muscles are also in bad shape, we might begin to leak urine if our bladder feels full. Loss of muscle and tissue tone in the pelvic cavity can also lead to a *prolapse*. This is when the organs in the pelvic cavity begin to drop because the muscles and tissues holding them in place have become slack and lost their elasticity. As they drop, they press on whatever is below them. The uterus, bladder or rectum can all bulge into the vagina.

REMEDIES

There are some exercises called Kegel Exercises (see p. 99) which can usually solve the stress incontinence and milder prolapse problems. However, like all weak muscles it has probably been a long slow decline in activity that has left them in a floppy unhealthy state, and so patience and perseverence will be required to exercise them back into a healthy working order.

If the prolapse is very severe or giving you problems, it is possible to have surgery either to tighten up the ligaments supporting things inside, or else to have a hysterectomy. However, you should certainly try the exercises first – and give them a genuine opportunity to work – before having anything so final as surgery unless it is absolutely necessary. And you might find it helpful to talk to The Hysterectomy Self Help and Support Group (see p.104).

SWEATS
See Flushes and Sweats.

SWOLLEN BREASTS, FEET, HANDS, STOMACH, etc
See Bloatedness.

TEARFULNESS
See Depression; Irritability.

TIREDNESS
See Exhaustion; Insomnia.

URINARY SYMPTOMS
See Stress Incontinence; Vaginal Changes.

VAGINAL CHANGES
Sometimes around the time of menopause, women experience varying degrees of vaginal dryness or soreness. The skin inside the vagina and around the vulva, or vaginal opening, becomes thin and less well lubricated. It can become itchy or sore – especially during sex if this includes penetration of the vagina. Sometimes the urethra and bladder are also affected and may become tender and sore, giving rise to pelvic distension (bloatedness) and urinary problems. Some women also experience dryness in their nose, and skin generally. Occasionally, the vaginal soreness can become serious as the lining of the vagina may begin to stick together and become extremely painful. Not enough research has been done on the subject to be able to say why this is, or who it affects. For example, it may be more of a problem where women have demanding sexual partners who require penetration as the only form of love-making. Or it may occur more with women who have less sexual activity and whose pelvic cavity and vagina are less exercised.

At present, little is known about who gets vaginal changes, the extent to which they get them, and what the other factors are in their lives that may contribute. All women have fluctuating hormones and lower levels of oestrogen in their bodies after the menopause, but not all women have vaginal changes. However, it is thought that, when women do experience vaginal changes, it is related to lower oestrogen levels circulating in the body. But, as we've said, far too little is known to be able to make definite statements.

REMEDIES

(1) If severe, hormone replacement therapy (HRT) can work wonders, either as tablets or as externally applied cream, but you will need to discuss HRT thoroughly with your doctor to see what risks may be involved for you, and, if you *do* have HRT, you should be closely and regularly monitored.

(2) If less severe, Vitamin E therapy can also work well, say 200–600 iu per day for two to three months (see under 'Flushes and Sweats' for suggested dose). But don't forget to have patience, as it will take three to five weeks for the Vitamin E to begin to affect your hormone production and body secretions.

(3) Ginseng is prescribed by doctors in Finland, Russia, China and Japan, and has been recommended by doctors in the USA and Britain. The problem with ginseng is finding a doctor who will take you and it seriously, and who is familiar with its use and knows the correct dosages for menopausal use. Also, health food shops sell a range of products which may or may not contain properly prepared and measured ginseng. (If you are interested, you could ask your local health food shop for leaflets or books.)

You should not take ginseng indefinitely: it mimics the hormone oestrogen, which is why it is effective for vaginal changes and flushes and sweats. But no-one knows if it also mimics the tendency of oestrogen to encourage the growth of cancerous cells or cysts. Furthermore, known side-effects include swollen and painful breasts and vaginal bleeding.

(4) *Kegel exercises* help to keep the vagina in a moist healthy condition. They also help to improve and maintain the pelvic organs, muscles, and tissues in good, elastic order. They can also increase sexual responsiveness and feelings. They are the exercises

taught to women after pregnancy to get the uterus and pelvic organs back into a good firm condition after the stretching of childbirth, but *they should be practised by all women regardless of childbearing as a basic part of pelvic health maintenance*! We consider that if young women were taught these exercises in adolescence far fewer gynaecological, menstrual and menopausal problems would occur later in life.

(a) Sit on the lavatory, comfortably, with thighs spread apart, straight in front of you parallel to the ground, feet flat on the floor (or a book or box if necessary).
(b) Start to pass water, and in the middle of the flow pull back on your muscles to stop the flow of urine. The muscle you use to successfully stop the flow is your pubococcygeus muscle.
(c) Release the muscle and allow the flow to finish properly.
(d) Repeat this each time you need to pass urine for a few days.

Once you have learnt to do this so that you can stop the flow completely in the middle and then start it again, you have isolated the necessary muscle, and you can now do the exercise anywhere, anytime, rather than only when you pass water. How about when you are doing the dishes or photocopying, sitting on the bus or in front of the TV!

You should start fairly gently so you don't make your muscle sore, say two to three pulls, four to six times a day, building up to 20 pulls or so six to eight times a day. Do them as fast as you can.

Alternatively, you could vary the exercise: try pulling in and holding for a few seconds each time. Or try pushing out on the same muscle as though you are pushing something out of your vagina (not to be confused with the pushing action used when emptying your bowels).

You could develop your own routine, but make sure you have located the right muscle and exercise it *regularly*!

(5) Swimming is another excellent exercise for the internal organs and muscles.
(6) Masturbation is also excellent exercise for the vagina and uterus, and can be an enjoyable experience for any woman whether in or out of a relationship. It also exercises the entire pelvic area.
(7) KY Jelly (obtainable from most chemists) helps with vaginal dryness and can be fun to use!

(8) If you are in a sexual relationship with a partner who continually favours penetration, suggest different forms of sexual activity. There are many good books around which you might like to get hold of for you both to read. But beware, there are also some very bad ones around too, that take a 'blame' the woman attitude! If your sexual relationship is a problem, consider getting in touch with a counsellor of some kind. If your doctor is sympathetic s/he may be able to suggest someone. Otherwise, try some of the agencies listed on pp. 106–7.

VITAMINS, MINERALS AND HERBAL REMEDIES

Vitamins and minerals are best taken in natural food as part of your daily diet. If you feel it may be necessary to supplement your intake, we would advise you to keep to the recommended doses listed on labels. We have occasionally suggested higher doses where these are specifically recommended for certain conditions. Avoid vitamins which are sold as 'megavitamins' – that is, vitamins sold in extremely high dose form. Herbal remedies contain active chemical substances which is why they can be effective. Because they are natural plants they are not necessarily harmless and should be used with the same caution as any other medication.

APPENDIX 1: USEFUL INFORMATION

This appendix is divided into sections and in each we list some books and organisations which can provide information or help.

OURSELVES

BOOKS

Our Bodies Ourselves, edited by Angela Phillips and Jill Rakusen (Penguin 1978).

A Woman In Your Own Right, by Ann Dickson (Quartet Books 1982).

In Our Own Hands, by Sheila Ernst and Lucy Goodison (Women's Press 1981).

Passages, by Gail Sheehy (Bantam Books 1976).

The Feminine Mystique, by Betty Friedan (Penguin 1963).

Pathfinders, by Gail Sheehy (Bantam Books 1982).

Ageing For Beginners, by Mary Stott (Basil Blackwell 1981).

Prime Time, by Helen Franks (Pan Books 1981).

Look Me In The Eye: Older Women Ageing and Ageism, by Barbara MacDonald with Cynthia Rich (Spinsters Ink, San Francisco 1984).

Women As Winners, by D. Jongeward and D. Scott (Addison Wesley 1981).

I'm O.K. You're O.K., by T. Harris (Pan 1973).

Spare Rib Older Women's Pack of back issues with relevant articles (£4 inc. p & p from Spare Rib, 27 Clerkenwell Close, London EC1, 01 – 253 9792).

HEALTH

Women's Health Information Centre (WHIC). An organisation whose aims are to:

(1) Make information on women's health available to women.
(2) Support self-help groups.
(3) Work for improvements in the health services for women.
(4) Publicise and campaign on women's health.
You can phone (01 – 251 6580) on Tuesdays and Thursdays 10 am to 4 pm or write enclosing an SAE to 52–54 Featherstone Street, London EC1.
Health Education Council (HEC), 78, New Oxford Street, London WC1A 1AH. Phone 01 – 631 0930, and in Scotland 031 – 447 8044. Self-help leaflets can be obtained from them on a wide range of health topics including: examining your breasts; cystitis; sickle cell anaemia; thrush; period pains; and pre-menstrual tension. The HEC is also producing a booklet on the menopause. Some publications are in Asian languages.

BOOKS

A Gentler Way with Cancer, by Brenda Kidman (Century Publishing, London 1983). Alternative approach to cancer.

Our Bodies Ourselves, edited by Angela Phillips and Jill Rakusen (Penguin 1978).

Womancare; a gynaecological guide to your body, by Lynda Medaras and Jane Patterson (Avon Books, NY 1981).

Self Treatment for Colitis, by Harry Clements (Thorsons 1978). Gives causes, and offers self-treatment based on nature cures.

Herbs for Constipation and other Bowel Disorders, by Nalda Gosling (Thorsons 1982).

Hysterectomy: What It's All About, by Nancy Duin and Wendy Savage, free, from Thames TV Help Programme, 149 Tottenham Court Road, London W1P 9LL.

Women On Hysterectomy, eds. Nicki Henriques and Ann Dickson (Thorsons 1986).

Menopause: A Self Help Care Manual, by Santa Fe Health Education Project (New Mexico, USA 1980). Available from Sisterwrite Bookshop (see below). Short readable booklet with guidelines for setting up and running a menopause self-help group.

Life Change, by Dr Barbara Evans (Pan 1984). Chapters 9, 10 and 11 give a good account of the pros and cons of HRT.

Stand Tall! The Informed Women's Guide to Preventing Osteo-

porosis, by M. Notelvitz and M. Ware (Triad, USA 1982). Explains how bones change and what osteoporosis is.
Menopause: A Positive Approach, by Rosetta Reitz (Unwin 1981). A good read, encourages women to spend more time taking care of themselves in the middle years. Provides helpful information on diet and nutrition.
Coping With Periods, by Diana Saunders (Chambers 1985).
Why Suffer? Periods and Their Problems, by Lynda Birke and Katy Gardner (Virago 1979).
Women and Migraine, by L. Goodison. Available c/o 7 St Marks Rise, London E8.
The Patient Patient: Women and Their Doctors, by Helen Roberts (Pandora 1985).
Patients' Rights (HMSO 1983) free from National Consumer Council, 18 Queen Annes Gate, London SW1 9HH.
For Her Own Good: 150 Years of the Expert's Advice to Women, by Barbara Ehrenreich and Deidre English (Pluto Press 1979).

CONTACTS

British Association of Cancer United Patients, 121–123 Charterhouse St, EC1 M61A (01 – 608 1785). Information and practical advice.
Women's National Cancer Control Campaign, 1 South Audley Street, London W1Y 5DQ (01 – 499 7532).
The Mastectomy Association, 26 Harrison Street, off Grays Inn Road, London WC1 5DQ (01 – 837 0908).
Endometriosis Society, 65 Holmdene Avenue, Herne Hill, London SE24 9LD. Voluntary self-help organisation.
Hysterectomy Self Help and Support Group, 'Rivendell', Warren Way, Lower Heswall, Wirral L10 9HV (051 – 342 3167).
Menopause Self-Help Groups. To see if there are any self-help groups in your area you could try these contacts. WHIC (see above), Health Centres or Clinics, Well Woman Clinics, Family Planning Clinics, Health Education Units (for all these contacts look in your local telephone directory), Mid-Life Centre, Birmingham Settlement, 318 Summer Lane, Birmingham B19 3RL (021 – 359 3562 Tuesdays and Thursdays).
Women and Migraine, c/o The Migraine Trust, 45 Great Ormond Street, London WC1 (01 – 278 2676).

The Patients' Association, Room 33, 18 Charing Cross Road, London WC2 (01 – 240 0671).

ALTERNATIVE AND COMPLEMENTARY MEDICINE

BOOKS
Alexander Principle, by Dr W. Barlow (Arrow Books 1975).

CONTACTS
British School of Shiatsu, 14 Brooklyn Road, Bath BA1 6TE (0225 – 331357).

The British Chiropractic Association, 5 First Avenue, Chelmsford, Essex CM1 1RX (0245 – 358487).

International Tai Ch'i Chuan Association, 40 Hillcroft Crescent, Wembley Park, London W9 (01 – 902 2351).

Bach Flower Remedies Limited, Mount Vernon, Sotwell, Wallingford, Oxon OX10 0PZ.

Bioenergetics, The Open Centre, 188 Old Street, London EC1 (01 – 586 4143).

Women's Natural Health Centre, c/o Kentish Town Women's Workshop, 169 Malden Road, Kentish Town, NW5 (01 – 267 5301); women's health generally – homeopathy, psychotherapy, osteopathy, acupuncture and herbalist counselling and self-help courses on alternative medicine. Phone between 9 and 10 am for appointment.

New Approaches In Cancer, c/o Seekers Trust, Addington Park, Maidstone ME19 5BL (0732 – 848336).

The British Acupuncture Association and Register, 34 Alderney Street, London SW1V 4EU (01 – 834 1012). Will tell you your nearest acupuncturist.

The British College of Naturopathy and Osteopathy, 6 Netherhall Gardens, London NW3 5RR (01 – 435 7830). Lists local practitioners.

British Homeopathic Association, 27a Devonshire Street, London W1N 1RJ. Lists local practitioners.

The British School of Osteopathy, 1–4 Suffolk Street, London SW1 4HG (01 – 839 2060).

Institute for Complementary Medicine, 21 Portland Place, London W1N 3AF (01 – 636 9543).

Royal Homeopathic Hospital, Great Ormond Street, London WC1N 3HR (01 – 837 3091).
Society of Teachers of the Alexander Technique, 10 London House, 266 Fulham Road, London SW10 9EL (01 – 351 0828).
Alexander Teaching Associates, 188 Old Street, London EC1 (01 – 250 3038).

BEREAVEMENT

BOOKS
The Courage to Grieve, by Judy Tatelbaum (Heinemann 1981).

CONTACTS
National Association for Widows, c/o Stafford District Voluntary Centre, Chell Road, Stafford ST1 2QA (0785 – 45465). Mrs Eileen Hunt. Ring for local groups or contact people.
Cruse, Cruse House, 126 Sheen Road, Surrey (01 – 940 4818). Counselling by phone or local contacts. Support for Widows.
MIND, 22 Harley Street, London W1 (01 – 637 0741). Referrals to organisations dealing with bereavement and psychological distress.
The Gay Bereavement Project (01 – 837 7324).

COUNSELLING, THERAPY AND SELF-DEVELOPMENT
CONTACTS
British Association of Counselling, 37A Sheep Street, Rugby VC21 3BX (0788 – 78328).
Northern Ireland Association for Counselling, 0232 – 226778.
Scottish Association for Counselling, 031 – 445 1851.
Family Welfare Association (several branches), 501 Kingsland Road, London E8 (01 – 254 6251).
Parents Anonymous, 01 – 668 4805. 24-hour counselling for women worried by the desire to abuse their children in moments of stress.

Rape Crisis Lines
London – 01 – 837 1600.
Cardiff – 0222 – 373 181.
Glasgow – 041 – 221 8448.
Leeds – 0532 – 440058.
24-hour counselling and advice for any woman of any age who has been raped, whether recently or in the past. Centres in 40 cities.

Women's Aid, national number 01 – 831 8581. Support and temporary refuge for women who are suffering in violent relationships – mental, physical or sexual abuse.

Incest Crisis, phone 01 – 890 4732.

Marriage Guidance Council, 76A New Cavendish Street, London W1 (01 – 580 1087). Free counselling service on any kind of relationship problems, not just marriage. Look in local directory for nearest contact person.

Women's Therapy Service
BRADFORD: c/o Bradford Council for Voluntary Services, 9 Southbrook Terrace, Bradford BD7 1AD.
BRISTOL: Women Therapists Network, Naomi Roberts (Bristol 556890).
LEEDS: c/o Leeds Council for Voluntary Services, 229 Woodhouse Lane, Leeds LS2 9LS.
MANCHESTER: Catherine Prior, 25 Turnbull Road, Manchester M13 0PZ (Manchester 224 7563).
NOTTINGHAM: 23 Rutland Road, West Bridgeford, Nottingham (Nottingham 812 798 evenings, or Sheffield 614 300 ansaphone).

Spare Rib Magazine, 27 Clerkenwell Close, London EC1 (01 – 253 9792). Available from newsagents or by subscription. 'Shortlist' section lists courses, workshops and conferences.

Women's Therapy Centre, 6 Manor Gardens, London N7 (01 – 263 6200/09). Send SAE for programme.

Pellin Centre, 43 Killyon Road, London SW8 (01 – 622 0148) for programme of workshops, courses and groups.

Redwood Women's Training Association, 83 Fordwych Road, London NW2 (01 – 452 9261). Assertiveness training and women's sexuality groups.

Southampton Women's Counselling and Therapy Service, 15 Harold Road, Shirley, Southampton.

Birmingham Women's Counselling and Therapy Centre, 43 Ladywood Middleway, Birmingham B16 8HA (021 – 455 8677).

DRUG DEPENDENCE OR PROBLEMS

BOOKS

The Tranquilliser Trap, by J. Melville (Fontana 1984).

That's Life Survey on Tranquillisers, by R. Lacey and S. Woodward (BBC Publications 1985).
Trouble with Tranquillisers (Release 1982) available from Release, 1 Elgin Avenue, London W9 3PR (01 – 603 8654).

CONTACTS

Tranx, 17 Peel Road, Wealdstone, Middlesex (01 – 427 2065). Self-help groups for tranquilliser users.
DAWN (Drugs, Alcoholism, Women Nationally), 146 Victoria St, London EC4.
Alcoholics Anonymous, phone 01 – 834 8202.
Standing Conference on Drug Abuse (SCODA), 1/4 Hatton Place, Hatton Gardens, London EC9N 8NO (01 – 430 2341).

DEPRESSION, STRESS AND RELAXATION

BOOKS AND CASSETTES

In Our Own Hands, by Sheila Ernst and Lucy Goodison (Women's Press 1981).
Dealing with Depression, by Kathy Nairne and Gerrilyn Smith (Women's Press 1984).
Unfinished Business, by M. Scarfe (Fontana 1981).
Depression: the way out of your prison, by Dorothy Rowe (RKP 1983).
Stress and Relaxation, by R. Madders (Martin Dunitz 1979).
Your Complete Stress Proofing Programme (including relaxation and meditation techniques), by Leon Chaitow (Thorsons 1984).
Ann Truefitt's Relaxation Tape, available from Endometriosis Society, 65 Holmdene Avenue, Herne Hill, London SE24 9LD.
Agoraphobia, for details of books and cassettes which can help, send SAE to Mrs J. Skene Keating, 16 Rivermead Court, Ranelagh Gardens, London SW6 3RT

CONTACTS

MIND, 22 Harley Street, London W1 (01 – 637 0741). Referrals to organisations dealing with bereavement and psychological distress. Advice on mental health rights.
Samaritans, 24-hour confidential help line. For local phone number look in telephone directory or ask exchange operator.

Relaxation for Living, Dunesk, 29 Burwood Park Road, Walton-on-Thames, Surrey KT12 5LH. An organisation whose aims are to promote the teaching of physical relaxation to combat the stress, strain, anxiety and tensions of modern life and to reduce fatigue. They produce leaflets entitled 'The Menopause', 'Male and Female', 'Better Breathing', 'A Relaxed Person', etc. They also run a correspondence course on relaxation.

EDUCATION, TRAINING AND FRESH STARTS

BOOKS
Second Chances: The Annual Guide to Adult Education and Training Opportunities, National Extension College, 18 Brookland Avenue, Cambridge CB2 2HN (0223 – 316644). The NEC also runs many correspondence courses.
It's never too late: A practical guide to continuing education for women of all ages, Joan Perkin (Impact Books 1984).
What Else Can A Secretary Do? (MSC 1984). Available from COIC Sales Dept., Freepost, Sheffield S1 4BR.

CONTACTS
The Open University, PO Box 49, Milton Keynes MK7 6AN. Offers a range of degree courses but also others to do with health, fitness and family welfare.
Equal Opportunities Commission, Overseas House, Quay Street, Manchester M3 3HN (061 – 833 9244). Free advice leaflets on a wide range of women's rights – e.g. pensions, tax, etc, as well as for women wanting to train for a new, or first, paid job or career in their middle years. For *Northern Ireland* you can obtain 'Start Again: Make a Fresh Start through Education and Training' from EOC, Lindsay House, Callender Street, Belfast 1.
Returners, National Advisory Centre for Careers for Women, Drayton House, 30 Gordon Street, London WC1H 0AX.
Workers Educational Association (WEA), 9 Upper Berkeley Street, London W1H 8BY (01 – 402 5608). Offers a wide range of classes and has many branches.
The Forum on the Rights of Elderly People to Education (FREE), Bernard Sunley House, 60 Pitcairn Road, Mitcham, Surrey CR4 3LL (01 – 640 5431). Brings together many organisations and

individuals wishing to promote all kinds of educational opportunities for older people. Produces a quarterly information bulletin giving details of local initiatives, research and publications.

The University of the Third Age, c/o The Executive Secretary, 6 Parkside Gardens, London SW19 5EY. Many local groups organise 'mutual aid' learning groups, some are connected to educational institutions. UTA involves older people in teaching as well as in learning, as researchers and organisers and it makes education available at home and in local communities. A manual on setting up new groups is available.

Further Education Colleges and Adult Education Institutes offer a wide range of part-time and full-time courses for adults. Some lead directly to higher education (degrees and diplomas) and may be called Access Courses. A variety of return to study, flexi-study and open learning courses are usually offered. None require 'O' Levels or formal qualifications.

Adult Residential Colleges. Offer 1 and 2 year courses. No formal entry requirements. Grant aided. Most offer qualifications which satisfy higher education requirements.

Hillcroft College (for women only), South Bank, Surbiton, Surrey KT6 6DF.

Coleg Harlech, Harlech, Gwynedd LL46 2PU.

Co-operative College run by and for the Co-operative Movement, Stanford Hall, Loughborough, Leicestershire LE12 5QR.

Fircroft College, Selly Oak, Birmingham B29 6LH.

Newbattle Abbey Adult College, Dalkeith, Midlothian.

Northern College, Wentworth Castle, Stainborough, Barnsley, South Yorkshire ST5 3ET.

Plater College (Catholic Workers' College), Pullens Lane, Oxford OX3 0DT.

Ruskin College, Oxford OX1 2HE.

HIGHER EDUCATION

All the above information concerns courses below degree level. However, if you want to proceed to degree or post-graduate level the following publications are helpful.

Opportunities in Higher Education for Mature Students, CNAA, 344–345 Grays Inn Road, London WC1X 8PB. Free.

Directory of First Degree and Diploma of Higher Education Courses and Directory of Post-graduate and Post-Experience Courses, CNAA, 344–345 Grays Inn Road, London WC1X 8PB. Free.

Grants to Students: A Brief Guide, applies to those ordinarily resident in England and Wales only. Room 2/11, Department of Education and Science, Elizabeth House, 39 York Road, London SE1 7PH and from Local Education Authorities. Free. For Scotland: SED, Awards Branch, Haymarket House, 7 Clifton Terrace, Edinburgh EH12 5DT.

Mature Students: a brief guide to university entrance, Committee of Vice Chancellors and Principals, 29 Tavistock Square, London WC1H 9EZ. Free.

Sponsorship offered to students by employers and professional bodies for first degrees, BTEC higher awards and comparable courses, available from careers services, public libraries or in cases of difficulty from Manpower Services Commission, Careers and Occupational Information Centre, Sales Department (CW), Moorfoot, Sheffield.

Mature Students – Entry to Higher Education, by Bell, Hamilton and Roderick (Longmans 1986).

EMPLOYMENT

BOOKS

Returners, by Elizabeth Dobbie, National Advisory Centre on Careers for Women.

It's Never Too Late, by Joan Perkin (Impact Books 1984).

How To Get A Job, by Marjorie Harris (Institute of Personnel Management 1983).

The Unemployment Handbook, National Extension College, 18 Brooklands Avenue, Cambridge CB2 2HN (0223 316644).

Life Doesn't End at UB40, produced by London Weekend Television (01 – 222 8070). Free.

The Survivor's Guide to Unemployment and Redundancy by J. Melville (Corgi 1981).

Creating your own Work, by M. Mason (Gresham Books 1983).

CONTACTS

National Advisory Centre on Careers for Women, Drayton House, 30 Gordon Street, London WC1H 0AX (01 – 380 0117). Publishes a book called *Returners* which describes career possibilities and the training needed for them.

Job Centres run by the Department of Employment. Information about jobs and WOW courses (Wider Opportunities for Women) run by the Manpower Services Commission or Training Opportunities Scheme courses (TOPS).

NOW (New Opportunities for Women). Short courses at many colleges to help women to return to work after a long gap. Check in local library or at your local college.

FOOD, DIET AND NUTRIENTS

BOOKS

Vitamins: What They Are and Why We Need Them, by Carol Hunter (Thorsons 1979).
Vitamin E, by Leonard Mervyn (Thorsons 1980).
Improving your Health with Calcium and Phosphorus, by Ruth Adams and Frank Murray (Larchmont Books, USA 1978) available from Thorsons Publications Limited, Dennington Estate, Wellingborough, Northants NN8 2RQ.

CONTACTS

The Vegetarian Society (UK) Ltd, Parkdale, Dunham Road, Altrincham, Cheshire WA14 4QG (for booklist).

LEISURE, SPORT AND EXERCISE

BOOKS

Sexual Health and Fitness for Women, by Kathryn Lance and Maria Agardy (Corgi 1983).
Yoga Self Taught, by Andre van Lysebeth (Union 1985).
Introduction to Hatha Yoga, by Margaret Perkins (Thorsons 1979).
Treat Your Own Back, by Robin McKenzie (Spinal Publications 1981).
Treat Your Own Neck, by Robin McKenzie (Spinal Publications 1983).
Banishing Backache, by H. Clements (Thorsons 1974).

CONTACTS

The Ramblers Association, 1–5 Wandsworth Road, London SW8. (01 – 582 6826).

The Keep Fit Association, 16 Upper Woburn Place, London WC1H oQG (01 – 387 4349).
The Sports Council, 16 Upper Woburn Place, London WC1H oQP (01 – 388 1277). There are nine regional offices of the Sports Council in different parts of England.

SEXUALITY

BOOKS
For Each Other, by L. Barbach (Corgi 1983).
For Ourselves, by A. Meulenbert (Sheba 1981).
Sexual Health and Fitness for Women, by Kathryn Lance and Maria Agardy (Corgi 1983).
Women's Experience of Sex, by Sheila Kitzinger, paperback (Penguin 1985).
The Hite Report by Shere Hite, particularly the chapter on older women (Dell, New York, revised 1981).
The Mirror Within, by Ann Dickson (Quartet Books 1985).
See also Chapter 12 in R. Reitz, *Menopause: A Positive Approach* (Unwin 1981).

CONTACTS
(SPOD) Sexual and Personal Relationships of the Disabled, 286 Camden Road, London N7 oBJ (01 – 607 8851).
Women Sexuality Groups, contact Redwood Women's Training Association, 83 Fordwych Road, London NW2 (01 – 452 9261).

SPECIAL NEEDS

BOOKS
Caring for an Elderly Relative, free fact sheet from Box 96, Central TV, Birmingham B1 2JL.
Who Cares for the Carers and *Caring for the Elderly and Handicapped*, both 1982 and free from National Council for Carers and their Elderly Dependents, 29 Chilworth Mews, London W2 3RG (01 – 262 1451).
Caring for the Elderly and Handicapped: Community Care Policies and Women's Lives, Equal Opportunities Commission, EOC 1982 (free).

CONTACTS

Association of Carers, Lilac House, Medway Homes, Balfour Road, Rochester, Kent (0634 – 813981). Unites carers in local groups to bring relief from extreme stress which can result from looking after someone. Supplies information on help available to carers.

The Association of Crossroads Care Attendant Schemes, 94A Coton Road, Rugby, Warwickshire CV24 4LN (0788 – 61536). Your local Social Services should have a list of what schemes are available in your own area (see phone book, listed under your Local Authority.)

GEMMA, BM Box 5700, London WC1V 6XX. A club for disabled/able-bodied lesbians to lessen the isolation caused by disability and offer access to feminist/lesbian literature.

Sisters against Disablement, c/o WRRIC, 52–54 Featherstone Street, London EC1 (01 – 251 6332).

(SPOD) Sexual and Personal Relationships of the Disabled, 286 Camden Road, London N7 0BJ (01 – 607 8851).

RADAR, 25 Mortimer Street, London W1 (01 – 637 5400). Advice, grants, holidays for people with disabilities.

Sportsline, phone 01 – 222 8000 for advice on sports/activities for women and facilities for women with disabilities.

British Sports Association for the Disabled, BSAD London Regional Officer, The Cottage, Tottenham Sports Centre, 703 High Road, London N17 (01 – 801 3136). Organises and gives information on sports activities for people with disabilities.

GLAD Directory of Clubs. You can order this listing of over 700 clubs for people with disabilities in Greater London from GLAD, 1 Thorpe Close, London W10 5XL.

WOMEN'S ORGANISATIONS AND FACILITIES

Equal Opportunities Commission, Overseas House, Quay Street, Manchester M3 3HN (061 – 833 9244). Free advice leaflets on a wide range of women's rights – e.g. pensions, tax, etc, as well as for women wanting to train for a new, or first, paid job or career in their middle years.

National Housewives Register, 245 Warwick Road, Solihull, West Midlands B92 7AH. Phone 021 – 706 1101. Local groups.

Women and Manual Trades (WAMT) is a group of women working in non-traditional manual jobs, who provide support, information and advice for other women who either work in manual trades or who are trying to get into these trades. The information they provide is practical, comprehensive and useful. WAMT publishes a *Yellow Pages of Training*. Women can either phone, write or visit the project. For more information contact WAMT, 52–54 Featherstone Street, London EC1 (01 – 251 9192).

National Federation of Women's Institute, 39 Eccleston Street, London SW1W 9NT (01 – 730 7212). National organisation which arranges sports, leisure and educational activities for women, particularly older women. Recently appointed a special sports officer to further these activities. Contact above for your local group.

The Women's Sport Foundation, c/o GES, Sheffield City Polytechnic, 51 Broomgrove Road, Sheffield S10. Aims to promote the interests of all women in and through sport, to increase sporting opportunities for women, to campaign against discrimination and to encourage women's confidence in starting new sporting activities. Information exchange. Write for details of local contacts.

Outdoor Woman, c/o A Woman's Place, Hungerford House, Victoria Embankment, London WC2. Women's group meet regularly to make outdoor pursuits accessible to all women and girls and to share organising, equipment and resources. Good contact point for meeting other women interested in particular sports. Write for details of meetings.

Local Women's Group, Contact WIRES, PO Box 20, Oxford (0865 – 240991).

Older Feminists Network, c/o AWP (A Woman's Place), Hungerford House, Victoria Embankment, London WC2 for nearest group and Newsletter (01 – 836 6081).

Older Lesbians Network, c/o London Friend, 274 Upper Street, London N1 (01 – 708 0234). Tuesdays and Thursdays 7.30 to 10.00 p.m.

National Union of Townswomen's Guilds, Chamber of Commerce House, 75 Harborne Road, Edgbaston, Birmingham B15 3DA. Provide a meeting ground for women of all ages. Helps members develop new interests. Local groups. Details from above address.

A Woman's Place, Hungerford House, Victoria Embankment, London WC2 (01 – 836 6081). Main central London women's liberation meeting place, has bookshop and meeting rooms.

LIBRARIES

Many local libraries now have a women's issues or women's studies section. If *your* library can't supply you with a book you want, ask them to get it on Inter-Library Loan for you.

BOOKSHOPS

For Bookshops outside London
Consult the 'Booksellers' section in *Spare Rib Diary* or ring *Spare Rib* (01 – 253 9792) and ask. Or ring Airlift Book Distributors (01 – 251 8608) and ask which bookshops in your area they distribute to.

Bookshops in London
Balham Food and Book Co-Op, 92 Balham High Road, London SW12.
Bush Books, 144 Shepherds Bush Centre, London W12.
Virago Bookshop, 34 Southampton Street, Covent Garden, London WC2.
Sisterwrite Bookshop, 190 Upper St, London N1 (01 – 226 9782).
Silver Moon Bookshop, 68 Charing Cross Rd, London WC2 (01 – 836 7906).
Owl Bookshop, 211 Kentish Town Road, London NW5.
Reading Matters, 10 Lymington Avenue, London N22.
Centreprise, 136–138 Kingsland High Road, Hackney, London E8 2NZ.
Booksplus, 23 Lewisham Way, London SE14.
Kilburn Bookshop, 8 Kilburn Bridge, Kilburn High Street, London NW6.
Compendium Bookshop, 234 Camden High Street, London NW1.
Village Books, 17 Shrubbery Road, London SW16.
The Bookplace, Peckham High Street, London SE15.
Websters Bookshop, 1063 Whitgift Centre, Croydon.

APPENDIX 2: MENSTRUAL CALENDAR

DAYS	1	2	3	4	5	6	7	8	9	10	11	12	13	14	15	16	17	18	19	20	21	22	23	24	25	26	27	28	29	30	31
MNTH																															
JAN																															
FEB																															
MAR																															
APR																															
MAY																															
JUN																															
JUL																															
AUG																															
SEP																															
OCT																															
NOV																															
DEC																															

This calendar is for keeping a record of when your periods begin to change.
Examples of entries you might want to make are:
PD – period due   P – period   NP – no period   F – flushes, sweats
H – headache   B – bloated feeling   I – irritable
BT – breast tenderness   S – swollen feet, legs, tummy

APPENDIX 3: MID-LIFE QUESTIONNAIRE

This questionnaire is to help you find out more about your self; it is divided into three sections:

Looking Back;   Life at Present;   Life Ahead.

How much detail you want to put in is up to you. You may like to do it by yourself or with a woman friend.

Its purpose is to get you *thinking* about your life now, and how you see it in the future, so that you can begin to plan changes if you feel the need.

If you decide to write out detailed answers to any of the questions, you will need to give yourself more space: how about using an exercise book as a sort of personal diary?

SECTION ONE: LOOKING BACK

(1)   What were the major, or most important events in your life when you were aged:

up to 10 . . . .
10–15   . . . . —
15–20   . . . .
20–25   . . . .
25–35   . . . .
35–45   . . . .
45–55   . . . .
etc.

Using the same system answer the following questions as well.

(2) What were your greatest 'ups' and successes?
(3) What were your worst 'downs' and disappointments?
(4) What were the biggest decisions you made?

(5) What were your interests and leisure hobbies?
(6) What were the turning points and major changes?
(7) What were the happiest times?
(8) What were the unhappiest times?
(9) What are your regrets/what would you have done differently?

SECTION TWO: LIFE AT PRESENT
(Put ticks where appropriate)

(1) What are your relationships like?

With your:	Good	Unsatis-factory	Do you want to change it?
Partner	......	......	......
Children	......	......	......
Relatives	......	......	......
Friends	......	......	......
Workmates	......	......	......
Employer/boss	......	......	......
Employees/juniors	......	......	......

Add in anyone else, or think of individual friends or relatives etc.

What are your personal aims and ambitions concerning:

(2) Education/training/work/career?

....
....
....

I haven't thought about it because I haven't had:

the time ......
the opportunity ......
any encouragement ......
the right kind of support ......

(Tick where appropriate or put down other things that you feel have prevented you.)

I am happy and satisfied with things the way they are:
Yes..../No....

I want to plan some changes here:
Yes..../No....

Using the same system, explore your aims and ambitions concerning the following as well:

(3) Leisure/interests/sports/hobbies/physical activity.

(4) Homelife/domestic set-up, arrangements, roles etc.

SECTION THREE: LIFE AHEAD

(1) Where do you want to be, and what do you want to be doing when you are aged:

35–40 ....
40–50 ....
50–60 ....
60–70 ....
and so on.

(2) Do you want, or need to make any changes now:

in relationships with others? ....
in personal ambitions? ....

(3) Do you want, or need to make plans now for your future aims and ambitions? If so, in which area of your life?

....
....

(4) How will you go about making them?

If you feel the need to make some changes in your life, we hope that this book will have provided you with some ideas: several chapters have been written with this aim in mind.

APPENDIX 4: CALCIUM IN SOME COMMON FOODS

Food	Amount presented as mg in 100 g (3½ oz) of food
Cheese:	
Cheddar	800
Cottage cheese	60
Danish Blue	580
Edam	740
Parmesan	1220
Processed	700
Spread	510
Fish:	
Boiled prawns	150
Salmon	93
Canned pilchards	300
Canned sardines	460–550
Fried sprats	620–710
Fried whitebait	860
Fish paste	280
Fruit:	
Figs, dried	280
Lemon, whole	110
Flour and baked foods:	
Bread (white or brown)	100
Hovis (UK)	150
Cake, sponge (fatless)	140
Flour, plain (cake)	130
Flour, self-raising	350
Soya flour	210–240
Wheat bran	110

Food	Amount presented as mg in 100 g (3½ oz) of food
Nuts (shelled weight):	
Almonds	250
Brazils	180
Sesame seeds	870
Vegetables:	
Haricot beans (navy)	180
Kidney beans	140
Broccoli	100
Chick peas	140
Greens (turnip, kale, collard, mustard)	98
Parsley	330
Spinach (boiled)	600
Watercress	220
Yoghourt, low-fat (145 ml/5 oz)	180
Milk (98 ml/3·53 fluid oz)	180

Canned fish are a rich source of calcium when they are the kind which include softened bones, like sardines. Self-raising flour seems richer in calcium, but this is because it contains added baking powder which has calcium in it. Milk is a good source, and taken as skimmed milk less fat will be included. Some foods are quite high in calcium content, like spinach and rhubarb, but they also contain oxalic acid which stops calcium being available, and they should therefore be eaten sparingly.

INDEX